SURVIVING LEUKEMIA

Hope for William

AMY DELAISSE

Surviving Leukemia
Hope for William

Copyright © 2015 Amanda Delaisse

Cover design by Sharron Blood/Dusk Meadow Design

Published in the United States of America

ISBN-10: 151430354X
ISBN-13: 978-1514303542

DEDICATION

This book is dedicated to our family and friends who worked tirelessly and sacrificed much for our family, and to the Hope for William community of friends who lifted us up to God, day and night through prayer. Together we moved a mountain and watched a miracle unfold.

And to the selfless stranger that shared her bone marrow so that my son would have a chance to live. As a mom there are no words that can adequately express my gratitude. You gave William the gift of LIFE! And you gave me the greatest gift of all; you gave me the gift of time! More time with my son, more time to talk, more time to watch him grow and mature into the future God has in store for him.

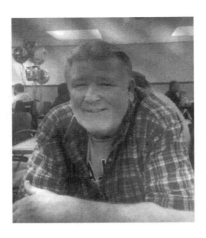

In memory of Gary Stephens
November 21, 1952-December 16, 2013

Gary, your death came so suddenly. I wasn't prepared for it. You were supposed to be okay. You made it to transplant. You were supposed to get better and we were supposed to have the big celebration barbeque back home. I just never imagined you wouldn't make it through. If I could ask God anything, I would ask him to give me just one more conversation with you. I would tell you that you were one of the greatest men I have ever met. You were so kind, so full of love and faith. I miss talking with you, I miss your infectious laugh and the way you walked into a room of strangers and within minutes knew everyone by name. I am honored that I got to know you, even for the brief time and I am honored that we got to fight this beast together. You helped give me strength and hope. And even though I feel like part of that passed away with you, I'm gonna keep fighting for now, but when my time comes, we are going to have that barbeque celebration in Heaven!
William

Still Here

You don't have to be here... to still be here.
You don't have to speak or laugh or pray here...
to still be heard here.
You don't have to wrap your arms around us here...
to still be felt here.
Your smile, your spirit, your prayers, your hugs
changed our world - indeed - they changed us.
You can never truly be gone
because your life still lives here, on and on
in every chemo treatment, in every fight we fight
in every "good morning," in every "good night."
And even though you've finished your race,
and you're there gazing upon our Savior's face
we know that every extra day we get
is probably 'cause you still ain't stopped praying for us yet.
That was just you... that IS you
beautiful, wonderful, amazing... you.
So you don't have to be here... to still be here.
No you don't have to be here... to still be here.
You don't have to be here... to still be here.

by Scott Sean White

PREFACE

On May 11, 2013 my twenty-year old son, William began coughing up blood. He was taken to the emergency room and diagnosed with pneumonia. After a week of antibiotics and rest, he was better and returned to work. A few weeks later, on June 5th he called me on his way to work.

He was having pain in his jaw that was so severe he was in tears. I had no idea what was going on, I thought perhaps it was a dental issue. By the next morning he was having heart attack symptoms and was rushed to the ER by ambulance.

At the hospital, a series of tests were ordered, including chest x-rays, contrast lung test, blood work and CT scans. All the while, no one was talking or giving us any answers. He was admitted into a room, so we knew "something" was going on but had no idea exactly what. The only thing the doctor said was his white cells were "funny shaped and out of whack." At 10:34 p.m. on June 6, 2013 the doctor gave us a diagnosis of leukemia, but he was still waiting on the results from the bone marrow biopsy to determine what kind and a treatment plan.

As I walked down the hallway toward William's room, I passed signs that read "Chemotherapy" and "Oncology." It still didn't register. I couldn't understand why they put him in a room on the cancer floor. It was a county hospital, so maybe it was the only available room they had? He didn't have cancer; it was just mono or the pneumonia returning. He *couldn't* have cancer!

When I walked into his room I saw a sign that read "Hematology Oncology," and the reality of the situation began to sink in. I knew hematology meant blood, and oncology meant cancer. That was the exact moment I realized leukemia was a blood cancer. The doctor walked into the room and handed me two booklets. One was about leukemia and the other was about chemotherapy. I just sat down and cried. How can this be? There wasn't time to fall apart, though. William was in a critical state. His cancer was advanced. His bone marrow was over 80% cancerous, and the cancer had penetrated into his central nervous system and was going to his brain. Chemo would need to be started immediately, or he would die within days.

I started searching for a book about leukemia that would help prepare me for what was coming, so I could also help prepare William. I knew chemo would make him sick, but I wanted to know more. What would help the nausea? What other side effects could he have? How can we make it more comfortable for him? I found several books on cancer, but most were for spiritual help, and I really wanted something that addressed the medical and physical side effects and progression of the disease. I was completely lost. I had no idea of what was coming and doctors were using terms I had never heard of.

My friend Kendra is a young cancer survivor, so I sent her a text with William's diagnosis. She set up a page for William on social media so I would have a way of updating several people at one time. My phone had been ringing off the hook with well-meaning friends and family wanting to know what was happening. I lost track of whom I had called and whom I hadn't. It was all so overwhelming!

As I made the posts on William's page, I tried to include

the physical effects of the chemo so people would understand exactly what he was going through. The battle is emotional, physical and spiritual, and I wanted to include all this on his page, to give people an understanding of what cancer really looks like. I tried to give an honest representation of what was happening to William in case someone out there was about to face the same journey. Sometimes, just knowing what is coming helps you prepare for it. As other cancer and transplant survivors found his page, they began sharing their experiences, and what helped them. We became a community, as people from all over the world joined and followed William, sharing their stories and cheering him on as he walked this path.

I am not a doctor. I am a cancer mom, a "Momcologist," if you will. Leukemia is a unique cancer. It has many types and subtypes. Even after helping my son through it, I still do not fully understand every aspect of it. Therefore, this book is not intended in any way to offer medical advice or take the place of your doctor's advice or treatment plan. This book might open up some ideas to discuss with your doctor, but always consult your doctor before trying anything new. There are very serious drug interactions that could put you or your loved one at serious risk. I have also included a glossary of terms at the end of the book. These are just very basic definitions of some of the acronyms, terms and words you may see while going through the book.

Not every cancer journey will be the same as ours because each person is unique, as is their illness. This is our experience, and these are my posts as I walked with my son on his cancer journey.

SURVIVING LEUKEMIA

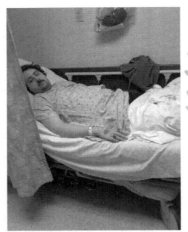

June 6

8:34 P.M. OK, I am starting to worry and cry now....I do not have a diagnosis but I have more information. William's white blood cell count is out of whack and they said they are shaped "funny." They need to run several more tests on him. Other things are not right but they didn't specify what "other things." They have not ruled out pneumonia again but are not saying too much until more tests are run. He is being admitted until they figure out what is going on because really, they just are not sure. Please pray for him.

9:27 P.M. I need any medical people to help me out. They have done blood tests, EKG and chest X-Rays on William. Dad just texted me that the doctor wants more blood tests and a contrast lung test. We don't have any clue what they are looking for, but here are my questions: 1.) Could this be related to his pneumonia last month? and 2.) Would this be a common test if looking for a heart attack? William went in with heart attack symptoms, so they were looking for that. Any takers on this one? I know I should wait for the doctors, but seriously...this is my child we're talking about here, and I am not that patient!

10:34 P.M. I can't even believe I am typing these words, but William has leukemia. We are waiting on a bone marrow biopsy to find out what kind and if it's fatal. He is getting a blood transfusion now, and we are waiting on doctors to discuss chemo. *How* is this possible? I know God is in control, but my heart hasn't quite caught up to my head, and when it's your child, it's harder to accept. I need some time to fall apart so I can pull myself back together for what lies ahead. I ask for non-stop prayers. Please don't stop praying for him.

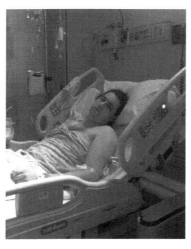

June 7

This has been the worst day of my life. *Leukemia* is the word every parent fears. As I walked down the hallway towards William's room, I passed signs that read "Chemotherapy" and "Oncology." I just kept thinking this can't be right. Why did they put him on the cancer floor? He can't have cancer. This has to be a mistake! I feel so helpless. I just want to *do* something, but I can't. I can't make him feel better. I can't even hug him because he can't tolerate the pressure and pain in his bones when anyone touches him in any way. This is my child and I can't comfort him in any way. He is scared. They put a PICC line in him today, to give him his chemo. I can't take this pain away; I can't make this all better. I am just helpless.

We do not have his bone marrow biopsy results yet, so I don't know what type of leukemia we are looking at, or even what stage he is in. So many of you have offered to be tested to see if you are a match, but I don't know yet if we are going to have to do that. I don't really know what is next, besides the obvious (chemo).

Right now, I have more questions than answers, but I just want to ask that everyone keeps William in your prayers and put him on prayer lists at your church, during your Bible studies – everywhere - anywhere. I still believe in the power of prayer and I know God is still on His throne. In Genesis, the angels asked Abraham "Is anything too wonderful for the Lord?" and I am holding on to that verse as my promise that God can do anything!

June 9

Thank you Kendra, for setting up the Hope for William page on Facebook. I will keep everyone updated as I have new information.

As you know by now, William has been diagnosed with leukemia. He was taken to the hospital on Thursday with heart attack symptoms and while they were trying to diagnose a heart attack, they found leukemia. We have all been blind-sided by this. We wondered if it was related to the pneumonia he had a couple of weeks ago, but the doctors have compared all the labs and assured me this is an acute leukemia and was not present at that time.

He is receiving blood transfusions daily at this time, either platelets or red blood cells. He seems to improve for a little while when he gets these. His first round of chemo through his PICC line will begin tonight. He has already had a small of chemo injected into his spine. He is getting two red cell transfusions now. They will wait an hour and start his chemo. The chemo treatment will last three days and he will be in the hospital for about four to six more weeks. They want to watch him and monitor his reactions to the chemo through the first two rounds. He will have a total of eight rounds. Then he will need a bone marrow transplant. The transplant will need to be done at MD Anderson, in Houston.

So many have asked how they can help right now and there are two ways to help. One is to go to Carter Blood Care and donate whole blood or platelets. It will help replenish what William is taking. I will call Carter tomorrow and set it up, where he gets credit for your donations. The next thing you can do is to register to be a bone marrow donor. William does not have a full sibling. He has a half-brother and half-sister but they are two years old and four years old, so they are not even old enough to be looked at as a possible donor. So they said our next best option is the national registry. His doctor said it is rare that the match will come from someone we know, therefore we have to literally move a mountain of people. William's match may be someone *you* know. Tell all your friends and family to sign up. We will be hosting drives to sign people up and I have some dear friends helping me do this, so more information will come soon.

Please be sure to pray for him. That is the most important thing you can do. I still believe God is in the business of answering prayers, and I believe He will heal my son. It will be a hard road with ups and downs. But in Genesis, when the angels came to tell Abraham he and Sarah would have a baby (and they were both very old), Sarah laughed to herself and the angels asked Abraham why she laughed and asked him "Is anything too wonderful for the Lord?" That question is my promise that God can do anything, and my "wonderful" is to heal my son.

Also post your messages to William, messages of hope and

encouragement, because in the days ahead, he will need them to keep his spirits lifted. He will begin feeling the effects of the chemo soon, and he will likely get worse before he gets better. He needs to know that so many people love him and are supporting him, and this will help him when he is in the valleys of his journey.

June 10

I think I am finally at the place where I have accepted the fact that I can't change William's situation, so I have to believe God has allowed it for some reason. I haven't really accepted the fact he has cancer, just the fact that I have no control to change it or do anything about it. I am not happy about it, by any means.

William is handling it very well, though. He asked me to bring the clippers tomorrow when I come see him and to go ahead and shave his head. This is going to be hard. I just love his curly hair. And it will probably be very different when it grows back. I saw a can koozie on the Internet tonight that said "Cancer Sucks," and I think he would appreciate that because I can see him saying that. He is one-third of the way through his first chemo treatment. This really does suck!

Thank you all for your words of encouragement for William. He has enjoyed me reading them to him. I need to ask a favor. Due to the fact that his immune system is so compromised, all objects coming into the room have to be disinfected. For this reason, flowers, balloons, and cards are not the best idea as they can harbor germs. Please use this site for now to post your well wishes. And before you visit, please avoid large crowds such as those in church, shopping malls, and movie theaters. If you have a fever or feel a little sick, please do not visit. He has no ability to fight off infections. Thank you all for understanding. Following these guidelines will help him in the best possible way.

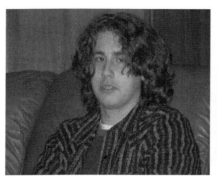 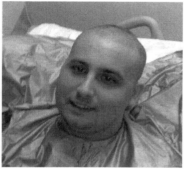

June 11

William is very tired. Please no visitors today. The doctors have ordered to limit to one visitor and one family member at a time. No exceptions. They reminded us that he has no ability of his own to fight germs, and he must remain as isolated as possible for the time being. The effects of the chemo have begun. They started this afternoon, so I would expect my next several posts on his Hope for William page will not carry good reports. The doctors are still waiting for his test results to come in. They said it is a difficult case, and have brought in some additional doctors to help. But he was hoping that by 5:00 p.m. today, we would have all the info, so I expect when his team comes in tomorrow morning, we will know exactly what we are dealing with.

The picture of William with hair is one of my all-time favorite "hair" pictures. It was taken right after James was born, so he would be sixteen. And if anyone is wondering, yes, I cried through most of the haircut today. Not because he was losing his hair, but because *this* wasn't supposed to happen. And I am kinda pissed that it has! I know there is a healing process, and I am still going through it. William said he wasn't going to let the cancer decide when he lost his hair; it was going to be on his terms.

I have to tell you the story of why his hair was long to begin with. When he was thirteen or fourteen, I wanted to give him a buzz cut. So we made a deal, that on the last day of school we would do it, and he had all summer to grow it back if he didn't like it. In turn, I would let him grow his hair back as long as he wanted to. He hated the buzz cut. Hated it (so did I)! So he let it grow...and grow...and grow. He kept his hair long for about five years. He wore it in a ponytail and straightened out his curls (I think just to irritate me). He finally cut it about a year ago and donated his locks to Locks of Love. He looks good, though, don't you think?

June 12

Today has been full of ups and downs. William's labs are finally in, and he has acute undifferentiated leukemia (AUL) with T-cell markers. This means he is showing both AML and ALL. His lead doctor said, "He is a rare bird." There isn't any good bone marrow left in him, so a bone marrow transplant is a must. Leukemia is a blood cancer, so it is different than other cancers. They don't measure its severity in stages; it is based on how many cancer cells are in the bone marrow (called blasts) and other "markers" that determine how severe, or high risk, it is.

Some good friends are helping to organize some bone marrow drives to help us find a match for William. They do want to get him in remission first, but we need to get started on finding his match. So information will be posted here once dates, times, and locations are settled.

William is feeling the effects of the chemo now. He is very nauseated, and he is having severe headaches. They are going to see if changing his medicines would help him. He is very weak and tired. Not the William most of us know. He doesn't eat much at all. I was excited he drank two-thirds of a Boost today, to be honest. He did get up and walk down the hallway and back to his room. He wears a hat because he is a little shy about being bald. And he has to wear a mask to protect him from germs if he leaves his room.

Between the Social Security Administration and MD Anderson, I have been buried under a mountain of paperwork and phone calls. The social worker at the hospital filed for disability for him and the Social Security Administration wants to see all his bank records and pay stubs for the last six months. William does everything electronic, and they will not accept copies. I have to get every single page notarized and supply supporting documents from his bank and employer that he cannot get access to original documents. I carry a file around with every scrap of evidence on William's life. I call it the Identity Theft Folder because it contains everything you would need to steal his identity. But it never fails that when I am at the hospital someone calls and needs a piece of information that is back at home. I now just carry it with me everywhere I go. I also learned never throw any piece of paper away. If you wrote something on it, keep it!

I have also applied for grants through Heroes for Children and Leukemia Texas. Both of these organizations have grants available to help with hospital bills and medical expenses. Since William doesn't have insurance, these grants will go a long way in helping.

Comment 5: This is so IMPORTANT!!! I was Never as sick as William, but please do him a favor and protect him. I lost my immune system and it is awful...putting one foot in front of the other is more than your body can handle. Everyone must think...it is all about William.

Comment 9: FaceTime or Skype is a great way to visit and not share germs!

Comment 13: YOU GO AMY! YOU KEEP EVERYONE STRAIGHT AND WILLIAM SAFE - HIS LIFE DEPENDS ON IT.

Comment 20: You don't know me, but my husband went through chemo for lymphoma almost 2 years ago. You'll get a lot of advice, so I won't offer much, but just want to encourage you to KEEP TRYING on the nausea meds. They may not be able to solve it completely, but something will help. After a few things that worked for a little while, then seemed to "wear off", we finally found a cocktail that kept the nausea at bay maybe 75% of the time. He could eat almost normally (the smell issue was a constant one) and, after dropping about 35 pounds very quickly, his weight stabilized for the last 2 months of his chemo and he was much more comfortable. Anyway, just a note to not just accept the nausea. There are a number of things he can try! Hang in there! Our family will pray for you all.

June 13

I really enjoyed visiting with William today. He was a little stronger, at least until the Neupogen shot in his stomach. That made him hurt, and he seemed unsteady on his feet afterward. But he took half a lap down the hall, and I know just doing that takes all he's got right now. He went back and laid down and had a good nap after. It's amazing, imagine it taking all the strength you have to walk the distance from your front door to your mailbox. That's about equivalent to the distance he can walk. I will be so glad when he gets stronger. I hate to see him struggle like this. And through all he is going through, he was worried about my dog! Linus was bitten by a snake yesterday. A copperhead, the vet thinks. Linus is doing fine but it makes me smile that in William's pain and misery, he tries to comfort me and give me advice. What a big heart!

Today is one week from when William was taken to the hospital. I still struggle with accepting this. I still have a hard time hearing the words *leukemia, cancer and chemo*. It is so hard to believe that your whole life can be turned upside down in a matter of just a few days. William was working and hanging out with his friends like a normal twenty-year old, and in a matter of days he is fighting for his life.

I asked him today how he feels about all this. He said he is okay. He is lonely, and he misses his room and his stuff. I know hangin' with your grandparents and parents isn't fun, and I can appreciate that. I reminded him that he will get stronger, and once he does, the doctors will lift some of the visitation restrictions. He seemed to understand that pretty well. I know it's hard for him!

His lead doctor said William is exactly where they hoped

he would be after his first round of chemo. His headache has finally subsided as well. Now they just give him a cocktail of drugs to help with the side effects and general pain. They also gave him a shot that will go to his bone marrow and help his white cells function normally. That's the Neupogen shot, and they are very painful!

I wish this was all he needed but it isn't the case. It will just help. The doctor said he doesn't have any healthy bone marrow in him, so the transplant will be essential. We are working to get the marrow drives set up now. They said to expect him to have good days and bad days and not to panic if his fever spikes again, because it probably will. He has to get up and walk a little each day to help prevent blood clots and that is hard for him, but he is a trooper. He ate better today than he has in over a week. Overall, it has been a better day. I know darker days are coming, but I am grateful for the good ones.

June 14

William is very sick right now. His fever has spiked, and he is very weak and can't eat. They think he may have an infection. They are giving him stronger antibiotics and a platelet transfusion now. The doctor said to have no visitors except the immediate family until further notice. Please, call all your prayer warriors now!

June 15

I am sitting next to William right now, and I just can't get my head around this. He looks pale. His lips are just the color of his skin, not pink. He is getting a blood transfusion now, which might help give him some color.

He had two platelet transfusions earlier today and will have another red blood cell transfusion after this one.

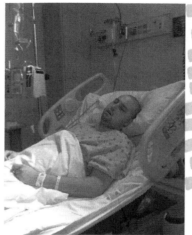

I thought just hearing his diagnosis was the worst day of my life, but to watch him go through this has been far worse. You can be told to expect bad days, but nothing really prepares you for it. He is hurting, and I can't do a thing for him. I just wish those good days would hurry up.

This is the post I made on my personal page last night after leaving the hospital. I was asked why I didn't post it here, and it was because it isn't very uplifting. I was reminded that falling apart is part of the healing process. I was asked to share this post on William's page:

"The last couple days have just downright sucked! William got some kind of infection and the doctors jumped through hoops to get it under control quickly, since an infection could turn deadly at this point. Today his fever spiked again and his doctor thinks he had a reaction to the blood transfusion. I just fell apart. We (his doctor and I) were in the hallway talking and I just lost it. I try to stay strong when I am with him, but I have never seen him so weak and frail! Dr. Ibrahim reminded me this is the worst part. The 10-14 days after chemo is the hardest. They were afraid the cancer was going to his brain so they gave him the strongest possible dose of chemo on his first round. With William's form of leukemia there is a 67% survival rate, which sounds great, unless it is YOUR child laying there! Then anything less than 100% is unacceptable. But Dr. Ibrahim said he truly felt William would make it through this. I know God is the ultimate Healer and statistics don't mean anything to Him! But I tell you, until you have to sit back and just watch your child fight to stay alive, you don't know how you will respond. Some days my faith is very weak and some days it is very strong. I just cling to the words "nothing is too wonderful for The Lord." I just kept rubbing his forehead today and telling him to get through these next few days. After that, the worst is over. Just fight like hell for a few more days! He said he could do it. He is tired and weak but he can do it!"

Comment 7: I wish I had words to make it better. I wish he didn't have to go thru this. I know there must be a purpose for this trial, and while you can't see it now, good will come from it. But all I want to do is find some way to fight it for him, as must you. I know you just want to scream at the cancer and demand it leave your son alone. It's not fair! Why William? Why your family! I don't have the answers. All I can do is pray and offer what support I can. But I do know beyond a doubt God will use your situation for good. Hang in there! All of you! And please let me know if I can help in any way.

June 16

Today was a better day. I got to sit with William for awhile this morning. When I first got there I noticed he looked better. His color was better, not so pale and gray. He was very tired, though. The blood transfusions took until 4:30 a.m. and because of the fevers they had to check his vitals every fifteen to thirty minutes. The Neupogen shots they gave him for the white blood cells are causing a lot of pain, which is normal so they increased his pain meds too. I hope it helps him sleep better. Kaitlyn, William's girlfriend, got to come see him today. I know that lifted his spirits a lot. He's been missing her. He ate pretty good today, too, which is always a good sign. Days like today that give me hope.

On my drive in this morning, I was thinking about faith and trusting God through this. I remembered when William was a very little fella, no more than four. We were shopping at Sam's, and I saw a beautiful old-fashioned roll top desk. I loved it, so William decided we needed to buy it. I explained that it was expensive and we would have to save the money for it, and just pray that they wouldn't sell out before we could. He walked up to the desk and rubbed his hands on it and said a little child like prayer that I can't even remember. But I will never forget what he did next. He turned to me, opened the second drawer on the left side, and said, "God said okay, and here is where I can keep my crayons."

Over the next several weeks, when we shopped at Sam's he would run to the desk and open that drawer and remind me that was his drawer for crayons. When we finally had enough to buy the desk, the floor model was the last one they had. We got the very desk he had prayed over... and a big box of crayons. I still have the desk.

We used to laugh and say William had a direct line to God. Maybe it was just his faith. He just believed God would always take care of everything, and he never doubted. I need some of that faith right now. Maybe we all do.

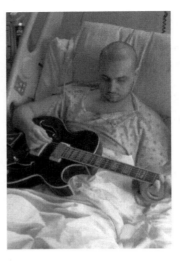

June 17

Today was a roller coaster ride! The ups were so great and the lows were so bad. This morning William looked fantastic. He was alert and talkative, and his color was close to normal. It was amazing to see him so much like his normal self. We even had a little "guitar therapy" early this morning. Then we took a short walk to the nurses' station and back to his room.

But around 1:00 p.m. it went south fast! The pain set in, and all he could do was lay in bed and moan. I just held his hand and reminded him to fight through the pain. About a year ago, I saw a breast cancer logo with "warrior wings" and I didn't quite understand the warrior part until now. William (and the others fighting cancer) really do have to fight like warriors. Some days it's the physical pain they fight, and other times it's an emotional fight.

June 18

William had a great night and has been fever free for two days! It is safe to allow visitors again! We still have to follow the same guidelines as before, only two at a time, etc. Be sure to call my sister, Kelly, to schedule a time if you want to visit him. She is making sure not too many people show up at one time, making sure everyone has a chance to see him.

If you plan to visit him, please be sure to avoid crowds as

much as possible for several days before your visit. This includes shopping malls, movie theaters, church, etc. He still has no ability to fight off illnesses and is very susceptible to catching anything "going around."

Also, if you would like to send him a card, you can mail it to him and my sister will take a picture and post it here on his page so he can see them. Since he can't have cards and stuff in his room, this is a great alternative, and all the cards will be kept for him for when he returns home. Some have also asked about gift cards. Right now, he is craving Subway sandwiches, Taco Cabana and Wendy's hamburgers. Chicken of any kind makes him sick, just the smell of it. He said the hospital food is awful. Dr. Rutherford, his lead doctor, teases him because we bring him food. She says he must be pretty darn special.

Speaking on behalf of the entire family, I want to thank you all so much for your continued prayers and words of encouragement. You are all helping keep William's spirits up, and ours as well. Keep praying, God is listening.

June 19

We have all heard the saying, "attitude is everything." I have to hand it to William; his attitude is pretty amazing right now. He shaved his head because he wasn't going to let the chemo take his hair. He was going to lose it on his terms. Through the headaches, body aches, dizziness, weakness, nosebleeds, itchy skin, nausea, throwing up, losing his hair, fever, blood transfusions, shots in the stomach...through all these issues, he still manages to find humor. Sometimes I wonder if he really understands just how serious this really is. But he does; he just *will not* let it defeat him and he will not wallow in self pity. He is a fighter, and I couldn't be more proud of him.

June 20

Today is two weeks. William says he feels like he has been in the hospital for months. We are in a "hurry up and wait" pattern right now. They will run more tests on him in a few days to make sure the chemo is working as they hoped. In the meantime, he just has to work through the side effects. He has had several nose bleeds today and his skin is just itching like crazy. The doctors said it is drying out from the chemo. I will miss seeing him tomorrow, since I have to run a lot of errands and get some paperwork ready for MD Anderson, where he will have the bone marrow transplant.

If you haven't already, please join the bone marrow registry, either online or in person at one of our drives. And do one more thing for me; once you register, be sure post to let William know. Encourage your friends to register too. Only God knows where his match is; we don't. We know his match is out there because "is anything too wonderful for the Lord?"

June 21

William had an okay day today. He is still hurting pretty badly, and the shots they give him in his stomach really make him hurt worse. His white blood cell count is up from zero, which is a small improvement. It is not quite where they hoped he would be, but it's an improvement. A small victory is still a victory! He will have to continue the shots to help raise the numbers and when they are better, he will do round two of chemo. He has another bone marrow biopsy this coming week. Pray for comfort for him for the coming week; he will need it. The shots and biopsy are both very painful.

June 22

Great news today! William's white cells took a big jump today to 1.7! They were very low yesterday, so the doctors were very encouraged by this. His doctors will continue to monitor the count daily. When the white count gets a little higher they will do another bone marrow biopsy, and then the second round of chemo. I never thought I would be excited about a round of chemo, but it means William is improving. For now, they are going to suspend the shots in the stomach and the antibiotics and just let his body work. The shots cause a lot of pain in his bones so this will also hopefully help alleviate some of his pain.

June 23

Today has been a rough day for William, both physically and emotionally. He is in excruciating pain in his feet, back and ribs. The pain meds are just not working, and he isn't getting relief. He is missing his pets, his room, his stuff, his strength and quite frankly...his life. He doesn't have the strength to walk ten feet today. He feels like a shell of who he once was. He is depressed and he is angry. And he feels guilty for being angry.

I just can't stand to see him like this. I told him all these emotions are normal and it's okay to be angry! There are some people on this site who are cancer survivors, so you know how he feels. What can I say to help him? What helped you get through the rough days?

Comment 2: All the emotions are normal. It is his

body and it feels like it is being taken away from him. Tomorrow will be a better day, it is ok to have a bad day every now and then, just do not allow yourself to dwell in the bad, because tomorrow maybe his best day yet. Nor sure if you are playing praise and worship music in his room but that is the only thing that got me through. Put on positive music...I have gone through chemo but not nearly what he is going through. I am praying for him and your family. Psalm 30:5 Weeping may endure for a night, but joy comes in the morning.

Comment 11: Debbie is so right....the bad days are usually worse than the worse day last week....but keep the faith and think positive and then all of a sudden....the good days when you do not feel as bad as the last bad day are more often and they last just as long as the horrible days....cuz right now the good days go by way too fast.

June 24

William had a better day today. Turns out, one of the night doctors changed his medicines without consulting his lead doctor. This is what caused the pain yesterday. The night doctor had adjusted the medicines to where they were pretty much ineffective. The night nurse tried her best to help but William pretty much just had to suffer most of the night. Early in the morning, as in around 3:30 a.m. to 4:00 a.m., they changed him back to where he should have been and he finally got some relief. My dad and I both talked with Dr. Ibrahim this morning and he handled it. We are pretty certain this won't happen again!

Tomorrow morning they will do another bone marrow

biopsy and then set the date for round two of chemo. With each round, they will inject some of the chemo into the spine to help protect the brain and make sure the cancer doesn't get into the brain.

So that's all the technical stuff. On a personal level, William is still a little angry and "edgy" that this is happening to him. The doctor said that for at least six months he will not be able to drive, work, eat out with friends, go to a movie theater - all those things twenty year-olds do. He will stay pretty much isolated at Mom and Dad's house, or our house. That will be a huge adjustment for him. He feels like he is losing himself. But I just remind him, it will only be a short time and then after he is in remission and gets his transplant, he will be able to get his normal life back.

I have finally reached the place where I truly believe William will survive this. I don't think I have truly accepted it. I still cry myself to sleep every night, and when I wake up in the morning, I have a heaviness in my heart. Most mornings when I wake up, I am still in disbelief that this is happening. The thought that my son may die haunts me. I watched the recording of him playing his guitar the other night, and showed it to his little brother and sister, and I thought to myself, *what if I lose him and I never get to hear him play again?* But somewhere deep inside, I feel that won't happen. I finally have faith that he will beat this. I still cry when I talk about it, I still can't believe words like *cancer, leukemia and chemo* are part of my daily life. I think most of us really think "this won't happen to MY child." I had thought that. But reality is, it can. And you can't prepare for it. You can never really prepare for this. But I also know that God is in control of everything. Even when you can't trace His Hands, trust His Heart.

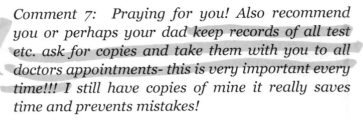

Comment 7: Praying for you! Also recommend you or perhaps your dad keep records of all test etc. ask for copies and take them with you to all doctors appointments- this is very important every time!!! I still have copies of mine it really saves time and prevents mistakes!

Comment 11: Amy, I remember you telling me about the night before William was born and how you felt God wrap his arms around you... He is here with you and your family now just like he was that night. And now He has the help of all of us, your friends and family that truly love ya'll and will be there and do everything we can to help until William is back on his feet again. And I have no doubt that the remarkable young man that you've raised will be with us for many, many more years to come. Love you girl!

June 25

It has been a rough couple of days, and today is no different. They did the bone marrow biopsy this morning and said they will get the results at the end of the week, but Dr. Ibrahim can already see some improvement over the first biopsy. The pain in his bones is still pretty intense and the biopsy is pretty painful in itself. He is battling depression right now, and I think it is from the pain. Round two of chemo will begin this week. I am ready for some more of those good days to come back. It breaks my heart to see him suffer and see him so down. I am hoping and praying tomorrow will be a better day for him.

June 26

We had a successful blood drive today at Mockingbird Station with Carter Blood Care. I felt so guilty for not being with William at the hospital, but I wanted to be at the blood drive to donate and to personally thank everyone who came to donate. My sister, Kelly made chocolate chip cookies and my sister-in-law, Kathi made brownies to pass out to everyone as well. I have donated blood many times but never truly understood how precious that donation really is until this happened to William. Your donations will mean the difference of life and death to so many people. You really are heroes. Thank you!

June 27

Round two of chemo began yesterday. So far, William is doing pretty well with the side effects, mainly nausea right now. What is left of his hair is starting to come out easily now. He had bald patches in his beard, so he shaved that today. He should complete this round by Sunday night and if they can get his medicines all switched to a pill form instead of an IV, and he doesn't get any infections or complications, he will be able to come home soon. He has to go back three times a week to have his blood checked, get transfusions, etc. He will be admitted for a week with each round of chemo, but at least he will be back home in his environment. He will be somewhat isolated at the house for the next six months. By then, I bet he will be pretty tired of his environment. ☺ One of his friends came and stayed the night with him so the family could rest at home, and they took a long walk. Actually they were looking for a Mr. Pibb and finally found one several floors away.

I really want to pause for a moment, and say how incredibly grateful I am to so many people who have helped us as we go through this. I know it is only one part of the journey, but we are overwhelmed at the outpouring of help we have received. Everyday life comes to a stop when something like this happens, or at least you feel like it does. Friends and family have helped us in so many ways...cooking, grocery shopping, watching James and Abbey, organizing blood drives and bone marrow drives, answering phone calls, taking the dog to the vet when he was bitten by the snake, making phone calls, sending cards, sending money to help with expenses, sending your words of encouragement and your prayers, staying with him overnight when we can't. Just saying "thank you" doesn't seem to adequately express how much we appreciate your help, but I hope you know that we (the whole family) are so humbled by the help we have received, and can honestly say we would not have been able to handle this without your help, love, support, encouragement and prayers.

June 28

William got to endure yet another lumbar puncture today. They are putting some of the chemo in his spinal column to help protect his brain, since the cancer was heading there early on. He is kind of getting tired of being poked in the back but he has a good attitude about it. He suggested they do a "connect the dots" pattern with the needle holes, in his initials...only William!

He is looking forward to coming home and sleeping on a real bed. He is pretty sick of the hospital right now. I don't blame him, it's been over three weeks now. We will be finding out pretty soon when he gets to come home. There will be several trips a week to the hospital for follow up care even after he gets to leave, and a trip to MD Anderson for an evaluation. But I am pretty sure the first week will be busy with getting the house ready and modified, watching him real close for signs of problems, and going on several trips to the hospital for check-ups and/or blood transfusions. I am actually a little nervous about him coming home. Right now he is surrounded with medical personnel at his beck and call. But I guess we will figure it out and learn what to look for.

I am still questioning WHY this happened. I don't think I will ever accept "We just don't know, there is no real pattern and it seems to hit at random" as an answer. While researching about leukemia I learned some interesting facts. Did you know over 35,000 new cases of leukemia will be diagnosed this year? And over 14,000 of those will not survive. The odds suck! The need for bone marrow donors is great, and the donors are few. With new technology, being a bone marrow donor is more like donating blood and not nearly as painful and invasive as it was a few years ago. We can't do anything about the number of new cases being diagnosed, but we *can* help reduce the death rate. Please consider joining the bone marrow registry and give these people a second chance at life. Trust me, if it was your child in need, wouldn't you move Heaven and earth to help him?

June 29

This round of chemo has been rough. When I got there today William just looked at me and said, "Mom, I am so tired." Then he rolled over and slept. His eyes are so weak today. They gave him a lot of medicine today with his chemo to help with the side effects, and another blood transfusion. Usually he perks up after getting blood, so

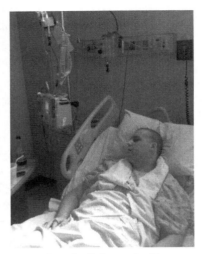 maybe tomorrow he will feel stronger. But right now he is suffering terribly! This chemo will last until 3:30 p.m. tomorrow afternoon (Sunday). It's a very hard chemo, nicknamed the Red Devil. Please help me pray for him through this.

William is normally strong and healthy. It's so unreal to see him weak like this. It's such a helpless feeling to sit back and have to watch and wait. But at the same time as we wait, we have seen God moving. It reminds me of the verse, "Be still and know that I am God." Knowing isn't the hard part, being still is!

June 30

William beat the Red Devil, and has been released from the hospital. Well, sort of, he still has to go back several times a week for check-ups, blood transfusions and small doses of chemo. He will only have to be admitted for the larger chemo treatments. But tonight he is happy to be back in his bed, and happy to see his dog Anna Belle!

This week we are running around picking up things he needs, medical equipment, groceries for his special diet (no foods prepared in the microwave), MD Anderson paperwork, etc. After this week, we should be in a pretty good routine providing he doesn't have any complications. We have to wear masks when we go shopping to avoid bringing germs back home to him. It's kind of scary not having the nurse staff there 24/7, but I guess we will figure it all out.

He is not out of the woods. He still has a very long journey ahead of him. We still have to find a bone marrow match for him. We will be hosting a community-wide bone marrow drive in Rowlett in the near future. We are having a planning meeting tonight at the Applebee's in Rowlett at 6:15 p.m. If you can help in any way, please join us at the meeting. If you aren't able to help with time, you may have the golden idea that we need! So please come. Amy Roseman with Delete Blood Cancer will be leading our meeting tonight, she said to come, "the more the *marrow-er!"*

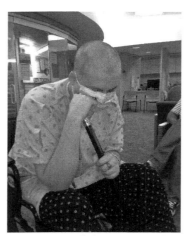

July 1

What a day - a long, miserable day! We spent the morning and early afternoon in the clinic doing William's transition appointment and lab work. Due to some confusion, no one seemed to know what was going on. William was about to pass out and was so weak he couldn't hold his head up, so after I started fussing and crying, finally we got help and he was seen. These are all new doctors and nurses, and I guess after the scene in the waiting room, someone went and got the doctor who has been seeing him while he was inpatient. It was so good to see Dr. Ibrahim coming up the hallway. It's amazing how much comfort is in a familiar face, especially when you are in a situation like this.

My favorite question of the day was when the nurse asked, "He sure does look awful tired. Has he had a chemo treatment recently?" Umm, YES...as in a twenty-four hour infusion of the Red Devil that ended at 2:30 p.m. yesterday! She was a little surprised he was released that soon after the Red Devil! But we have been assured the mix-up that caused today's chaos will not happen again.

After taking a nap when he got back home, William felt better, other than having some severe nausea. I think I may get some Tootsie Roll pops for him to see if that helps. James climbed up in bed with him, but Abbey is still a little nervous. I think William's bald head scares her a little. She's only two so she really doesn't have an understanding of what is happening. James is just so excited that his big brother will be at his birthday party (if William feels up to it). My two boys share a love of snakes. James was so excited to tell me that William is going to teach him all about snakes when he feels better. Let me just say I am not ready for another pet snake (so don't go there, William).

Thank you to the folks who came out and donated blood today in Rowlett. And to those who worked at the Celebrate Freedom Booth yesterday, all day in the hot sun. One hundred fifty-six people signed up on the bone marrow registry.

July 2

About eighteen years ago, when William was two years old, I saw a news story about donating bone marrow to save the lives of people's lives with leukemia. I remember thinking, "What would I do if anything like that happened to my baby?" I called the number and got some information to sign up on the registry, but I never followed through with signing up. There was always something to do and I kept pushing back until finally I just forgot about it. Back then, it wasn't as easy as swabbing your cheek and mailing it back in.

Now, here I am, a desperate mom praying to find a match for William. I can't help but wonder how many millions of other people did the same thing I did. You wanted to do it and had every good intention, but "life" happened and eventually you just forgot about it.

I found out there are around 11,000 people currently searching for a match on the registry. Friends, the time is now. If these people don't find a match, *life* for them won't happen. Over 14,000 people will die from Leukemia this year. Those people aren't just a number. They are someone's son, daughter, mother, father, sister, brother. They mean the world to someone, just like William means the world to me!

The donation process is not as painful and invasive as it used to be. Now it is more like giving blood. If you are pregnant and don't plan on banking your baby's cord, did you know you can donate the cord for stem cell transplants to save a patient with leukemia? If you are 18-55 years old, in good general health and with a body mass index less than 40, you can register. It can be done at one of our drives or by mail. Visit www.deletebloodcancer.org or www.bethematch.org for more information.

Now that you know...act! You might be the difference between life or death.

July 3

William has had a couple of pretty good days. He still has the nausea, but he is in less pain and able to get up and take short walks around the house. Today, the Neupogen shots in the stomach start back up. Those really hurt, and it makes his bones hurt so I am grateful he has had two fairly uneventful days to gain some strength. He has had some friends come visit and that helps lift the spirits. Thank you to everyone for continuing to go through his Aunt Kelly to schedule visits. It helps him not get over-tired and we still have to adhere to the strict guidelines from his doctor on how many can come, their illnesses, etc.

We are looking for a venue to host the big community-wide bone marrow drive in Rowlett. Once we have a place, we can set a date but it will be in about three weeks. We do have a booth at the Fireworks on Main tomorrow, so if you are close by don't wait. Go on over and get swabbed. If you are able to help with the drive coming up in a few weeks, or have a venue we can use, send an email to hope4william@gmail.com. We will need about thirty volunteers.

We have submitted paperwork for MD Anderson, and hope to hear soon when we can take him for an evaluation. Keep praying, he is far from okay and still has many difficult months ahead, and we still have to find his match to get his transplant.

July 4

Abbey is finally warming up and not as nervous about William being bald. It helps that he played the guitar for them. Both James and Abbey love to hear him play. When William was baby, I used to sing "Hush, Little Baby" to him. It was his song. When we found out a little brother was on the way, I told William I had to find a special song for James because "Hush, Little Baby" was already taken. I decided on "You Are My Sunshine" and William learned to play it. When James was fussy, William would play for James to help calm him down. Right now, James loves to sit next to William in the bed (and play with his cobra walking cane).

The bone marrow drive is still going on in Rowlett, so I don't have the totals yet, but they have been pretty busy since about 5:00 p.m. William was excited to hear it was going well. We still have two more drives coming up! July 13 in Lancaster on Historic Town Square and we are working on a venue to host a community-wide event in the Rowlett area, details still pending.

Keep those prayers coming. Chemo tomorrow, blood tests to determine if William needs another blood transfusion, nausea, pain - it's still tough. He gets up and walks around quite a bit but it wears him out quickly.

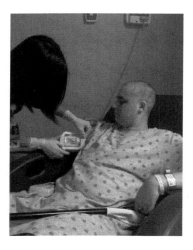

July 5

The chemo today went pretty quickly. Afterward the nurse changed William's PICC line dressing. That's what you see on his arm. The tube goes into his arm and across his chest and stops right before his heart. If I saw this on a stranger, I would be okay. But the fact that it is in my son kind of nauseates me. Not that it's gross, it's just that my son has to have it. He is scheduled for a blood transfusion on Tuesday. His numbers are getting low again. So we are on "fever watch" this weekend. Praying we have an uneventful weekend and no trip to the ER.

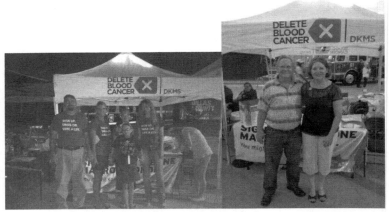

I want to give a shout out to some pretty amazing people: Uncle Billy, Aunt Kathi, Kasey, Mitzi, Avin, Deborah and Jerry. They have volunteered in three bone marrow drive booths in five days. All outside, in our Texas heat, and have added 284 more people to the Bone Marrow Registry. Look at their pictures. That is what a HERO looks like.

July 6

William is hanging in there, very tired and pale. On Tuesday he has a blood transfusion scheduled. Hopefully that will help him. He is on day four of the painful Neupogen shots, six more to go. Then he has another bone marrow biopsy and round three of chemo. It seems like when he gets over one hurdle, another one is right there before him. He has to fight his own way, but his fight is our fight too. We fight in other ways. We have to stay positive for him, keep telling him, "Just get through this phase. Just fight through it then you can rest." And let me tell you, when you see someone you love suffer so much, it is very hard to be positive. I still have melt-down days, and today was one. Some days I am just so freaking mad that William is going through this. I want to know WHY, I want to blame someone! I just kept telling God how angry I am and I kept being reminded of the verse "For I know the plans I have for you..." I wish He would let me have a sneak peek at those plans because right now I am just so angry!

> Comment 9: Can offer prayers, hope, empathy for you and William not from cancer but similar in severity. You probably already know this but small things really help your focus. They are keys to his health too. You're helping his mood by getting this off your chest so you can function better. I don't know you personally but you have many friends and supporters, some like me who have been where at times you can't see the forest for the trees even if you are doing a good job. Take care

July 7

Today was a really good day. We had James' birthday party and in between the birthday fun, I had the chance to sit down and talk with William. I have tried to make sure he doesn't see me fall apart, but we talked about it a little today, and I asked him if he is mad or wonders why it happened to him. He said not really. Maybe next time I am about to have a melt-down, I should talk to him.

He is just looking forward to getting to remission and past the transplant and getting his life back and being healthy again. He is also looking forward to growing his hair long again when his chemo is over. He misses his hair. I can understand that. He said when he can grow it out, he is going "Willie Nelson long" so be prepared.

It amazes me how strong he is. Even when he is physically weak, he is mentally and emotionally strong.

July 8
We received word that William didn't qualify for Social Security Disability and they are reviewing his case for SSI. That, however, they said can take until October 23 to make a determination. We are going to be doing some fundraisers in the very near future to help raise money for his medical expenses.

Petsmart (where William worked), and several friends and family have given money to help cover some of these expenses, and we have had many requests from people who also want to help. We want you to know how much we appreciate your prayers and your gifts.

July 9
William ended up getting two units of blood today, so it was a long day. But he needed it. He started getting some color after the first unit and "pinking up" nicely by the end of the second bag. He said he felt stronger afterward, even though he was a little tired from being out all day. More labs and check-ups on Friday and Monday, and then they will do another bone marrow aspiration and set the date to admit him back into the hospital for round three of chemo.

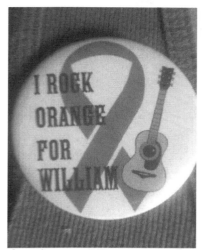

His nausea is a little better, but he is having some horrendous heartburn now. And he has developed a nasty cough, but they said his lungs are clear so it's just something we need to keep an eye on. He goes in for check-ups every few days so that won't be a problem.

Aunt Kelly has been busy. Check out her handiwork on the picture. We are squaring up details on a big blood and bone marrow drive that's coming up very soon. I will post details once they are all finalized, but plan on reserving July 28 if you are in the Garland/Rowlett/Dallas area. This will be fun!

July 10

William is so much stronger today after his blood transfusion yesterday. All day long, I have thought about the verse "For the life of every living thing is in the blood" (Lev. 17:11 New English Translation). The difference in his color, his energy and even his voice is amazing. I don't even know at this point how many units he has had, but I am so thankful to all the donors out there. One blood donation will save three lives. I never knew how precious those donations were until this happened. His need for blood will be ongoing as we continue this process so I want to encourage everyone to keep giving blood. Carter Blood Care has over one thousand requests for blood every day.

July 11

Well, we hit a bit of a rough patch today. William overdid it a little yesterday, and he is in a lot of pain today. It's so hard because he wants to do so much more than his body will allow him to right now. The doctors said he will get stronger as he goes through chemo and gets toward the end of his treatments, but this is still the beginning. I think on the days he feels better, he forgets to pace himself. He has another appointment with lab work tomorrow to check his blood and see if he needs another transfusion. We are just praying for a restful night tonight. Clinic days are long and hard on him too.

July 12

Today was another hard one for William, at least in the beginning. He had his doctor appointment and was low on potassium, so they fixed that. When he got home we talked for a while. He said the pain he feels is like nothing else he has ever felt. It's deep within him, he said he feels like his bones are in a trash compactor and are being crushed. I can't even begin to imagine what he goes through. Next week will be another bone marrow biopsy and then they will set the date for chemo round three. A silver lining though: they temporarily suspended the painful stomach shots, at least until Monday when they can re-check his numbers. That may help the bone crushing pain.

Tomorrow will be a very busy day. We have two consecutive bone marrow drives. The first is at Lake Pointe Church in Rockwall from 8:00 a.m. to 1:00 p.m., and there will be a Carter Blood Care bus at this location. A second bone marrow drive will be in Lancaster at Portal Comics on Historic Town Square from 10:00 a.m. to 2:00 p.m.

Now, the big news of the day. We are so thankful right now. The Hella Temple in Garland is going to allow us to use their large ballroom for a benefit for William on Sunday, July 28th. Plus, the Jimmy Jones Band is donating their talent and time to help us too. We have a space! We have a band! Now it's all falling into place. More details to come, but mark your calendar, tell your friends and plan to come. We need about thirty volunteers too, so let us know if you can help.

William hopes he can make it to the benefit concert, even if it is just for a short time. I honestly don't know if his doctor will allow it, just because of his compromised immune system. But he plans on asking anyway. He will have to wear a mask, and no hugs. He is moved that so many people are working so hard and giving so much of their time and resources to help him. You are really helping to keep his spirits up, even on the bad days. You are all so very much appreciated!

July 13

William had a good day, and we had two bone marrow drives today. Fox 4 news came to the one in Lancaster and did a piece on the news about William's search for a match. It aired at 5:00 p.m. and again at 9:00 p.m. Did anyone catch it? I hope many people will see it and step up to register. With a 1 in 20,000 chance of a match, we need as many registered as possible.

Starting next week, we will begin to work on the benefit concert for July 28. We will have fliers to pass to local businesses and yard signs. We need volunteers to help before and during the event so be sure to let us know if you can help and to get a yard sign. You can email us at hope4william@gmail.com.

Praying tomorrow will be another good day for William with lots of rest, so he is ready for his clinic appointments this week . On Monday he has labs and Thursday is another bone marrow biopsy (and those hurt).

July 14

Today was a day of reflection. Maybe it was the weather, 73 for a high and rainy in mid July is unheard of in Texas. I kept thinking about what has happened to us in the last five weeks. When something like this happens, it feels like your entire world stops. You don't have time to cook, grocery shop, clean your house, and return phone calls or anything else. But while you walk around in a stupor, life does continue. Before you know it, you are out of milk, toilet paper and clean clothes, and those simple things seem like the biggest stresses in the world.

Within the first days of hearing the news about William some wonderful people were there to help us. Kendra set up the Hope for William page and organized a blood drive. The first night, my neighbor Kim ran over and brought dinner and started organizing a bone marrow drive. She checked in to see if we needed groceries several times. My sister-in-law, Kathi cooked meals and grocery shopped for us and for my parents, in addition, she and my brother and their kids have worked several of the bone marrow drives in the hot sun. My mother-in-law cooked countless meals for us. We would come from the hospital and dinner was ready and hot. My friend Mitzi has been an incredible help at all the bone marrow drives. She works the entire crowd out in the hot sun all day.

So many others have helped in so many ways, Kyle, Phyllis, Kaitlyn, Deborah and Robby. So many people have come and stood by us to give us strength and hope during the hardest times we have ever had to face. Even people who have never met William or my family have sent cards and words of hope and encouragement. The kindness I have been shown by other has humbled me more than I can even express. I hope I didn't leave anyone out. I truly appreciate every person, every card, every call, every text and especially every prayer and every hug. I would not have the strength to watch my son go through this without such a wonderful support system.

July 15

After a very long doctor appointment today, William is pretty tired. This Thursday he will do the bone marrow biopsy to see if the chemo treatments are working as planned. Once those results are in, he will be admitted back into the hospital for the third round of chemo, likely staying about a week. I don't know if the Red Devil will be part of his next treatment. Either way, Red Devil or not, it is still chemo. So start lifting those prayers up for good results on the biopsy and strength for the coming treatment. Even with medicines to help with the side effects, it is still very hard to watch him go through the treatments and side effects.

July 16

Fox 4 news came out today and interviewed William about his leukemia and his hopes of finding a match. They let me know that because of the game tonight, the producers are holding William's story for tomorrow night, so watch for it tomorrow at 9:00 p.m. We are so grateful to have the opportunity to raise awareness of the bone marrow donation process. Over 14,000 people will die this year of leukemia, and they don't have to. With more people on the registry, more matches can be made and more lives can be saved. I am sure we will find William's match too!

William is very tired this evening, after a full day. He is resting well and getting ready for his biopsy on Thursday. Hopefully tomorrow will be another restful day for him because Thursday will be challenging.

Yard signs for the bone marrow drive/benefit on July 28 will be in Friday. Please send an email to hope4william@gmail.com if you would like to have one, and if you would like to volunteer. We are about to hit the road running, getting the word out. The more people who attend this event and join the registry, the better chance we have to find William's match. He is my son, he is everything to me. Please help me give him a second chance at life. Invite everyone you know to this event. Like his page, share his story. Don't wait. People with blood cancers are dying every day because their match wasn't found in time.

July 18

I have an amazing story to share with you tonight. I received this just a few minutes ago. I cried all the way through her story. I see it from the parents' perspective. How they must have rejoiced when they got the call. Elicia is a hero, and here is her story, in her own words:

"In March of 2009, I received a letter from the National Bone Marrow registry informing me that I am a match to a

10 month old little boy; a little boy who needed my bone marrow to live a healthy happy life. I put the letter aside for about a month or so. After thinking about it, and praying a countless amount of hours and talking to everyone I knew asking them what I should do. I knew it was destined for me to help save this little boys LIFE. I then contacted the Registry with a definite "YES" for my answer. I then went to do a consultation with the Medical Director from the collection facility on 06/23/09 and at that point I had to do a physical exam which was also performed on 06/23/09. It seemed like once a week before the surgery Carter Blood Care was collecting my blood to make sure I was still in good shape to have the surgery. Once I was all done with the test I went about 2 weeks before the big day. I stayed at the hospital the night before because I had to be there at 5am, July 17, 2009 was the big day me and my husband got up and walked down stairs to the hospital the whole way down there me and my husband where praying not only for me but for the little boy as well. I am not even going to lie I was scared but I kept telling myself the pain that I am going to be in for a week does not even come close to the pain this little boy and his family have gone throw in this short time of this CHILD life. He has not even had a chance to live his life. In a letter I got it said this child is very lucky to have found someone like me who was willing to help save his life. Without this transplant the patient would have not had HOPE for long-term survival of this disease with is WISKOTT ALDRICH SYNDROME. After the surgery my life changed for the better I have a new outlook on LIFE. On 6/17/10 I got the Bone Marrow Ribbon tattooed on my left wrist I did this is honor of the child because I am not able to meet him and his family so in some way to me the tattoo make me feel connected to him and his family. I also got the tattoo to helped spread the word of being a Bone Marrow Donner I am truly blessed to

have given this little boy and his family a second chance of LIFE. I would like to say thanks to Carter Blood Care and Be the Match for giving me a chance to help a child live a long healthy life."

Because the little boy that Elicia helped was under three, she had to do the more invasive procedure where they go in through the hip bone and take the marrow. In 80% of the cases, you can do stem cells through the arm, similar to giving platelets.

Elicia, thank you for stepping up, thank you for putting your fears aside. I know the parents of that baby thank you every day of his life. You are an inspiration and I hope your words help others who are nervous about giving a commitment like this.

> *Comment 2: That is so exciting! We hear stories of people who need a transplant. But to hear of someone who donated bone marrow and how it enriched their life! God is pretty wonderful. I would love to see a picture of the tattoo.*

> *Comment 9: You are a true unsung hero hopefully this will help others in their decision to make a difference in someone's life .*

> *Comment 18: Elicia, thank you for being so generous and selfless and a true hero. The family of the little boy that you saved will think of you every day of their life, you will always have extra prayers in your corner!! I can't even begin to tell you how it feels to be on the receiving end (my son received his cells 3/21/13). It is overwhelming and emotional beyond words. You saved that child as much as a firefighter pulling someone from a*

burning building or pushing someone out of the way of an oncoming car. Don't ever downplay the difference you have made in the family of that child...you are a wonderful person, thank you for deciding to donate!

July 19

William is not looking forward to going back to the hospital for his third round of chemo. Let's be honest, it's chemo and it sucks! He said he is going crazy being stuck in the house and wants a road trip, and doctors and hospital visits don't count. He still can't go anywhere without his doctor's approval, and that just isn't happening right now since his immune system is still too compromised. He will go back into the hospital Monday and stay for about a week. After his chemo, he really won't feel much like doing anything for several days. He is getting up and walking around the house with the help of his cane, but that's really all he can do right now. He looks paler today than yesterday, which is usually an indication that it is getting time for another blood transfusion. I know that when he goes in Monday, they will check all that and take care of him.

I spent the day in Rowlett and Garland, passing out signs and flyers to the local businesses about the Bone Marrow and Blood Drive on July 28. Every business I approached allowed me to hang a poster or leave a stack of flyers for the event. I was just taken back by how loving and compassionate everyone was.

I am also very excited to confirm that the Red Cross will be at our event on July 28, taking whole blood donations. I know a lot of folks are afraid of needles, and even one of

William's friends told me she was, but for him she is donating. That's the spirit Crystal! For those who are nervous about needles, fret not, you can do this. Just enjoy the music and be sure to tell the person doing the procedure about your fears, they are great to help you. Some other things you can do to prepare are to eat a big lunch and drink lots of water. Do not drink coffee, tea or soda because they dehydrate you. But drink a lot of plain water. It will help you fill up the bag faster. I am serious, especially in this heat, plan to drink at least 32 ounces of water before you arrive. We have a goal for 45 blood donations! Crystal has already promised her blood so we need 44 more!

Also, if you are not able to give blood due to being out of the country or some other reason for disqualification, it does not mean you can't sign up for the bone marrow registry. There are different qualifiers for blood and bone marrow. There will be lots of people to help answer any questions you may have for either. So come on out and help in every way possible. William and thousands more are depending on everyday heroes like you.

July 20

William doesn't feel very good today. He is very tired and doesn't feel like getting up much. I am just hoping and praying for rest as he prepares to start his third round of chemo. Praying for no infections between now and then, and that everything will go smoothly at the hospital during the admittance process. This is all new territory for us, so we don't know what to expect.

We still have twenty-four yard signs for the event on July

28. If you have a high traffic area where you would like to place a sign, send an email to hope4william@gmail.com. We will be very busy this week with William back in the hospital and preparing for the event, so please plan to go by Mom and Dad's and pick up your signs and fliers. Kelly will work with you to make sure they are ready for you and give you the address, (hasn't she been great?).

When you place your signs, be sure to follow your city's regulations on where to place them. If you don't, most cities will remove them and throw them away. In most cities, you must place the sign behind the sidewalk. Avoid the grassy area between the curb and the sidewalk; it's usually a city easement. Please be sure not to block the view of traffic when you place them.

Be sure to invite your friends and family to this event on July 28. We need to add as many people to the registry as possible to help find William's match, and he hopes to help others as well, by finding more than just his match. We have a goal of 45 blood donors too. I have donated blood for a long time, but I have never really understood how important it was until I watched life come back into William as he received his transfusions. I tease him when he gets really pale; I tell him he must be getting a quart low again. But in reality, the donated blood of strangers has kept my son alive for six weeks. He would not be here without those donors. We will also be raising money for William's medical expenses and travel expenses to MD Anderson. There will be something for everyone.

July 21

William is even paler today than yesterday and he is very tired. I am actually relieved he will be going back in to the hospital tomorrow. Dr. Mom's (that's me) guess is that he is getting pretty low on blood again, and needs another transfusion. I know they will check his numbers at the hospital and take very good care of him. Tomorrow I hope to sit with his doctor and find out exactly what type of leukemia he has (AML, ALL or both), if the chemo treatments are working as planned and just a general update as to how we are now in comparison to when we started. I know William is not looking forward to the coming week, so please keep him in your prayers. The chemo treatments are very hard on him, even with the medications to help with the side effects. Thank you all for your continued support, encouragement and prayers.

Fox 4 called me, and William's story is going to air today at 5:00 p.m. and 9:00 p.m. Be sure to tune in!

July 22

William is grateful to finally have a bed after seven hours of waiting. What a long day! The hospital said they had a room ready this morning so we headed up. It was not the case. They were waiting for discharge papers for another patient and it took a long time. They tried to temporarily put him in a room with someone who had *unknown infections* and puss oozing from him. We pitched a fit, since he was about to get chemo and it lowers ability to fight infections. You just can't take those kind of risks with a neutropenic patient. So we waited in a semi-isolated family waiting room until William's room was ready. But he is in and settled now.

Dr. Mom was wrong, his blood counts were a little low but still okay, he was low on potassium. They started that IV and will start his chemo tonight at 9:00 p.m. He was pretty tired but we did get a little good news. This round of chemo will not include the Red Devil. He was very relieved. He is getting a couple different chemos this time, Methotrexate and ARA-C. From preliminary results of his bone marrow biopsy, it appears the chemo is working. There is definite improvement. That was great news! Keep those prayer coming, God is answering.

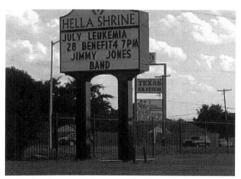

July 23

The sign is up at the Hella Temple. Yay! If you plan on volunteering to help, be sure to sign up. I have had several people ask if they need to schedule an appointment to give blood or to sign up on the bone marrow registry. The short answer is no. Just come on by anytime from 4:00 p.m. to 7:00 p.m. and we will gladly take your blood and/or your cheek swab with or without an appointment. And remember there are different qualifiers for blood and bone marrow. If you can't do one, you may still be able to do the other, be sure to ask. We are there to help.

I just spoke with Dr. Ibrahim and he said William's official diagnosis is acute undifferentiated leukemia. In layman's terms he said William has markers of two kinds of leukemia, AML and ALL. The chemo is working and the biopsy shows definite improvement. He was very pleased with how William has responded to the chemo. They did a spinal tap today but we don't have those results yet. William is doing okay so far with this round. He completes one chemo tonight and then another will start immediately afterward. Hopefully he will continue to do well throughout this treatment.

July 24

I have a lot of great news to share today. First, your prayers are being heard and answered. William is doing very well in this round of chemo; he hasn't even had to ask for nausea medications. His doctor approved him to come to the event on July 28 as long as he wears a mask and gloves and no "bro-fists," handshakes, hugs or kisses. I know that's hard but we still have to protect him from germs and illnesses, but he really wanted to come so he is very happy right now. It was a great spirit booster.

We also have a date for our appointment at MD Anderson now. We are MDA bound! This is great news. We will be doing all the preliminary tests and prep for his transplant. Once he goes into remission, and we have a match, they will want to act quickly for the transplant. Remission is only part of the battle because without the transplant, his leukemia will return and with no match, he will have to continue chemo until one is found. Please pray his perfect match is found quickly (and of course for remission and safe travels).

July 25

No visitors tonight or tomorrow, please. William is not well and needs to rest. Thank you for understanding. William is home from the hospital and happy to be in his own bed, but he is very tired and not feeling well. He has another clinic appointment tomorrow. No rest for the weary! I know he is looking forward to attending the event Sunday, so hopefully he can rest on Saturday.

July 27

About to call it a night. Busy day getting ready for the big event tomorrow. William feels better but is still fighting nausea, which is normal from his chemo. I am hoping he will feel up to making a short visit tomorrow. The event starts at 4:00 p.m., but the Red Cross will be set up to start at 3:00 p.m. for blood donations.

July 28

See you today at the Bone Marrow /Blood Drive and Fundraiser. It's from 4:00 p.m. to 7:00 p.m., but the Red Cross will be ready at 3:00 p.m. If you are donating blood, eat a hearty breakfast and lunch and drink lots of water so you are well hydrated. No special prep is needed for the bone marrow swab. The Jimmy Jones Band starts at 5:00 p.m. Come on over and save a life today!

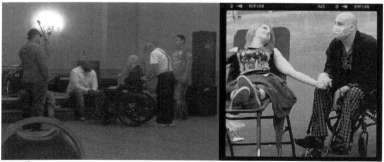

July 29

Yesterday's event was fabulous! We ended up with 44

blood donations and 78 people joined the bone marrow registry. The line was long to donate blood, but no one seemed to mind. William especially enjoyed meeting the band, and they are making plans to get together and have a mini jam session when William is better. He is really looking forward to that!

William's cousin Daniel also put word out to his unit about William, and 115 soldiers stepped up to donate blood. GO ARMY!

July 30

I am very happy to report that William has had a couple pretty good days. I am so thankful to God for those good days. We head to MD Anderson in a little over a week. He will have to endure more tests, but we will also get more answers. Everyone keeps telling me about the amazing work being done at MDA, I am just excited we are almost there. William isn't looking forward to having to go through all the tests again, but he is looking forward to being healthy again.

July 31

If you're following William's page and you're not on the National Bone Marrow registry, we need to talk. I have just heard of another leukemia patient passing. She was waiting on her match. That makes three in the last seven days that I have heard about. ALL OF THEM WERE WAITING ON A MATCH!

Trust me, if it was your loved one, you would be on the registry! One day it might be. Please, please, please get on the National Bone Marrow Registry. You can order a free kit at www.deletebloodcancer.org

I was driving today, and just thinking. I began to worry again about "What happens if there is no match?" and about future relapses, and just questioning *why* this has happened to William. But I suddenly began to think about the names of God and what they mean:

Jehovah Shammah - The Lord is present
Jehovah Rapha - The Lord our healer
Jehovah Jireh - The Lord will provide
Jehovah Yahweh - God's divine salvation
Alpha and Omega - the Beginning and the End, the First and the Last

I was reminded of who God is and what He can do. In His own words, "Behold I am Jehovah, the God of all flesh. Is there anything too hard for Me?" Jeremiah 32:27

No, it doesn't answer *why,* but it assures me that William is in bigger and more capable hands than mine, or even his doctors'. It gives me peace that God is bigger than cancer. It gives me hope.

August 1

10:26 a.m. Please stop now and pray for William. He went to his out-patient clinic appointment this morning and he is being admitted to the hospital. His hemoglobin level has dropped to 5, and he is very sick. I will have more of an update in a few hours, once he is stable.

1:35 p.m. William has had a platelet transfusion and is getting a red blood transfusion right now, and will have one more after this one. They have him knocked out right now so he can rest. 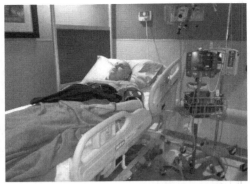 His red blood cell count and platelet counts were very low and his white count is almost zero. They have decided not to admit him, but due to the extremely low counts, we are back on fever watch and have to be extremely cautious for infections. We will be here for a long time and they will check his blood again after the next transfusion, before releasing him. Keep those prayers coming, he still needs them.

9:14 p.m. William is home, exhausted. Eleven hours in clinic, one platelet, two red blood transfusions and an overall minimal improvement in his numbers. His pulse was still high, but they felt it was alright to send him home with strict instructions. He just wants to rest, and has requested no visitors for a couple of days. He will be back on Monday, providing he doesn't have to make an ER trip over the weekend. This is evidently the nature of the beast with leukemia. My heart literally aches for him; there is just nothing I can do to ease his pain and discomfort. I have never felt so helpless. This is a horrible cancer!

August 3

7:52a.m. William was taken by ambulance to the hospital just a few minutes ago. He got up and wasn't able to feel his legs and fell, and his fever is over 100 right now. I will update more once I have more information, but please lift him up to God in prayer right now.

2:20p.m. Here is a quick update. William is in an isolated ICU unit of the ER. They will be admitting him and are getting a room ready for him. However, he is not stable enough to move from the ground floor to the 7th floor at this time. He has a designated doctor and nurse to stay with him constantly. The doctor was giving the nurse instructions and she snapped her head and told him, "I am NOT going to let him die!" He needs your prayers. He is on his second red blood transfusion and will also need a platelet transfusion after the reds. He is showing slight improvement. We are still waiting on results of his chest x-ray. More later...

7:40 p.m. William is stable and has been moved to a room. Still very pale and very tired. They are monitoring him very closely. He will get one, maybe two platelets today. They will check him tomorrow to see if he needs more red blood. The fever has come down a little but he is on some mighty strong antibiotics and they are looking for an infection. This has been an overwhelming day! William is so tired and we (the care givers) are emotionally spent.

August 4

William received two more red blood transfusions today. His platelet and white counts have come up but the red isn't responding very well, so we expect more red blood transfusions tomorrow. His fever has come down and is only slight now, but there is overall improvement. He was even cracking jokes earlier. One of the chemos he took in his last hospital stay, the ARA-C, is notorious for making blood levels drop, and its side effects peak on days ten to fourteen. That is why his hemoglobin and platelet levels dropped so drastically, and are staying low. We are not quite past the fourteen days yet. I really wish someone would have pointed out this is a common side effect of this particular chemo so we would have been a little better prepared.

I was thinking today on the way home about how great William's attitude still is. He hasn't been overly bitter or angry and he hasn't complained. That's incredible to me. One of his biggest disappointments in this was the day he realized he will never be allowed to donate blood again or be on the marrow registry himself.

I want to issue everyone a challenge. Tomorrow when you return to work, go to your HR person or whoever the decision making person is, and ask if you can hold a company-wide Swab Party. It literally takes about four minutes to sign up and swab to join the registry and potentially save lives. 14,000 people will die this year from leukemia, and roughly 11,000 of those are waiting on a match. Three died last week that I heard about, and they were all waiting to find their match. Imagine if this was your child. Wouldn't you do anything? If you will ask, and get the approval, I will put you in contact with someone who will help you. It's easy and quick and can be the difference in life or death for so many people. Please partner with us to help make sure no one ever goes without a match.

August 5

Grandpa stayed with William last night, and he called me this morning with an update. William's numbers have taken a leap into the safe zone and are holding. He is stronger. He can stand but is still pretty wobbly on his feet. They are taking him for some heart tests right now. They discovered a heart murmur, which is not a huge shock. When he was five he had a nasty bout with Scarlett Fever and I was told at any time he could develop a murmur. But they wanted to err on the side of caution and just make sure his heart has not sustained any damage in the last several days.

It is really good news, all the way around. I am preparing for our trip to MDA, and at this point they feel he will only get stronger throughout this week and will have no issues making the trip to Houston. This week, pray for continued strength and safe travels. Our first appointment at MDA is Monday morning, August 12.

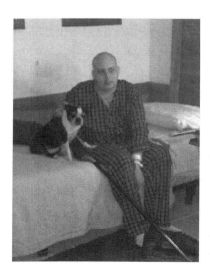

August 6

William is resting comfortably at home. He looks better than he has in over a week. His lips are actually pink again; before they were so pale they blended in with his face. He is up walking (with his cane) a little at a time. But he is stronger and better, and it's the little victories that make us so happy.

I wanted to stop and once again thank everyone who has helped us. From meals, to hosting bone marrow drives to financial donations, everything. I have been amazed and humbled at the outpouring of help and support we have received. I am way behind on thank you cards, but I want you all to know we would not have been able to handle this without your support, encouragement and prayers. I honestly don't have the word to truly express how grateful we are.

August 7

"Don't quit! Keep fighting through this!" That's what I told William two months ago when this terrible journey began for him. And he has. He has fought physical and emotional pain that most of us will never have to endure. He still has a long, hard road ahead of him, but I trust God will give him the strength to keep fighting.

But I want to tell you don't quit too. Don't quit praying, don't quit believing, don't quit donating blood and don't quit talking to people about the bone marrow registry. You see, thousands of cancer patients need blood to survive. Today I talked to a lady whose child had one hundred fifty blood transfusions by the time they got through their transplant. The need doesn't stop, so please keep giving.

I keep saying over 11,000 people will die, just this year while waiting for their match. Some of those people are in remission, but with this type of blood cancer, remission doesn't mean healed. In most cases, you have to continue chemo until you have a transplant, and the body can only withstand so much chemo. Talk to your friends and encourage them to join the registry. The only way to increase those odds is to add folks to the registry. Don't quit. People need you. The need will never end until there is a cure for cancer.

August 8

William had a good check-up today at his clinic appointment. His blood levels are good and holding nicely. He should be in good condition to make the trip to Houston this weekend. Now it's time to get ready. I have been making my list of questions.

Here is an interesting fact I learned about the transplant process: right now William's blood type is A- and he suffers from terrible seasonal allergies from December to February. After his transplant, he will adopt the donor's blood type (which could be different than his) and he will lose his current allergies and adopt his donor's seasonal and/or food allergies (if he/she has any). That's amazing!

August 9

Not much of an update today. Overall a quiet day, no emergencies. William got some much needed rest and I spent the day getting ready for the trip.

Pray for a match and pray for remission. But remember, in William's case remission doesn't mean healed, it's only the first step for the transplant. He has to be in remission to do the transplant, but he will have to continue those horrible chemo rounds until he has a donor. But we know God is in control, and before He formed William in the womb, He knew him (Jeremiah 1:5). So I believe He knew this would happen and He formed a match for him too.

August 10

William and I leave tomorrow for Houston, and the next phase of his journey. There, he will be "typed" and the search for a donor will begin. I will continue to update while we are away. We found out today that William does qualify for SSI. They denied Disability because you need a 10 year work history to qualify. With him only being 20, he doesn't have the 10 years so he will receive SSI instead. It isn't much but it will allow him to continue making his car payments (even though he can't drive), and it automatically qualifies him for Medicaid.

I want to ask for prayers for a little 6 year old boy and his family. His name is Aidan and he has Acute Myeloid Leukemia (AML). He has fought for so long, but it appears he will lose his battle very soon. Please pray for peace for his family as they say good-bye. Little Aidan will no longer be in pain, "And God will wipe away every tear from their eyes; there shall be no more death, nor sorrow, nor crying; and there shall be no more pain, for the former things have passed away." (Rev.21:4 NKJV). Please just pray.

August 11
According to his mother's post, The Lord took Aidan home just after midnight. Please pray for this grieving family.

We are here, just outside of Houston, staying with the sweetest family in the world. Tomorrow will be a very busy day full of appointments, consultations and orientations. William made the trip fairly well; he is very tired and sore right now. He said his bones feel like they have all been bruised. He felt like that this morning before leaving, so at least I know it wasn't the car ride (or my driving) that made him feel that way. We are both nervously looking forward to tomorrow; we have our list of questions ready. It will be a great day--I can just feel it!

Things were moving right along as planned. Countless people told me I had to get William to MD Anderson Cancer Center for treatment, and we were finally there. "It's a place of miracles," they would say. I felt like there was finally light at the end of a very long and dark tunnel.

But we were about to learn cancer doesn't play by the rules.

August 12

Well, today was a mix of good news and bad news. The bad news first, we were told to expect William to be in remission, but that does not appear to be the case. While we were registering, William felt his neck and he found his lymph node "chain" is back. He also has a swollen and sore lymph node in his armpit.

Dr. Alvarado, his leukemia doctor said the last bone marrow biopsy was clear but it appears the cancer cells are in the lymph nodes. He ordered some extra tests tomorrow and possibly a biopsy as well. Dr. Alvarado was surprised since William has endured some extremely strong chemo and he should not have any active cancer cells in him. He said it could be a very aggressive cancer and will require an even more aggressive chemo.

This quite frankly sucks and I am down-hearted right now. As I pushed him around the hospital in his wheelchair, I just cried. I have learned to cry silently so he doesn't know. I don't want to scare him. I keep telling myself the tests have not been run and this is speculation until we have the test results, which could be a few days. But in my heart, I know it's true. I knew the minute I felt his neck.

So what could possibly be the good news? Well, if he had a match now and went to transplant with active cancer cells, he would have had an over 80% chance of getting his cancer back. So by this "chain" coming back, it triggered more in-depth testing to be done, and they can make sure all the cancer cells are gone before we go to transplant.

Tomorrow will be an even longer day than today. William is very tired and will need a lot of rest tonight to get ready for tomorrow. It's not the good news we were hoping to hear, and it opens up a lot of new questions. But we will take it one day at a time. I was also "typed" today to see if I am at least a half-match. If there is not a full or near-full match for William, they will see if I am a close enough match with which to do something. It will be weeks before we start exploring these avenues because first he must be in remission. Please keep the prayers coming for remission, continued protection, and for strength for William to be able to tolerate the chemo side effects. Thank you for your continued prayers!

August 13

We are here for a twelve hour day of testing. William is already tired from yesterday. We understand it's a necessary evil so the doctors know exactly what they are dealing with, but it's still very hard on him. To be honest, I was hoping that when we got here to MDA, they would tell us there has been a terrible mistake and William was misdiagnosed. I was hoping to hear he didn't have cancer. But yesterday when I felt the lymph node chain on his neck, my heart dropped and I felt like the wind had been knocked out of me. Maybe I have just been in denial; I mean it just doesn't seem real that this is happening to my son! I kept asking the doctors back home if there is any way they were wrong on his diagnosis and they kept assuring me they were not. But I still kept looking for a way out; I just can't wrap my mind around this.

August 14

Yesterday was long and hard, and they had to postpone one of his tests. We are hoping to get it done on Thursday. We have no appointments today, so it will be a day of rest for William. I woke him up for his morning meds and then he fell back asleep immediately. The test they postponed is a PET scan. It shows active cancer cells, and they decided instead of doing a regular CT scan on his lymph nodes, they would do a full body PET scan so they can see where the active cancer cells are, and better determine a treatment for him.

I have new questions to ask, and have re-asked some of the old ones. After discovering the lymph nodes Monday, I feel like we are at Day Zero again. But I realize William is at the best possible place for his care. His doctors here are looking at everything, running every possible test, taking all my questions and exploring every angle. It is possible that our diagnosis may change once all the data is in. He is due for his next round of chemo but they really want to get a better idea of what type of leukemia he has before administering any chemo.

It looks like we will go home for the weekend and be back on Monday morning. We expect Monday to have a better idea of what we are dealing with and I expect him to be admitted for chemo next week. But everything changes daily so we will see.

August 15

The PET scan has been postponed until Monday (hopefully). Right now, William has a pneumonia pocket in his right lung which appears to be an active infection. They gave him a very strong antibiotic and since he is not symptomatic they did say it was ok to go home this weekend. He will stay on the antibiotic and return to MDA on Monday. Then he will meet his leukemia specialist, do the scan and be admitted for round 4 of chemo. But the great news of the day is that his bone marrow biopsy shows no sign of active cancer cells! Once we figure out the lymph node issue, we will have a clearer picture but it looks good right now. It will be a few weeks before we know if he has a match. Don't quit! Keep signing people up on the registry.

August 16

Please pray for William, this is taking an emotional toll on him.

> Comment 9: *This type of fight takes an emotional toll on everyone in the family... therefore, my prayers are for all that this touches and William. May our Father wrap His loving arms around each of you and give you peace and continued courage. Those of us that have trod this path understand and care deeply......*

August 17

Some days, hope is all you have. Thank you all for your encouraging words to William and those of us who are his caregivers. Some days are easier to get through than others, some days the exhaustion just gets the better of you. It's easy on those days to focus only on the bad news. But then you get a card, a text, a call or a message and someone encourages you and suddenly you have the strength to continue. Just knowing so many are praying for William increases my faith and my hope. Thank you all!

August 18

I am getting the oil changed, tires rotated, etc. Then we head out this afternoon, back to Houston. William's first appointment is at 6:30 a.m. on Monday. They are doing a

CT scan to look at the nymph nodes and pneumonia pocket in his lung. Then after a day of appointments, we will find out when he will be admitted for round four of chemo. Do keep praying, he will have to fight the Red Devil this round (which will be a further beating on his emotional state).

August 19

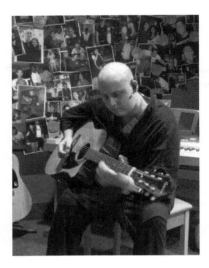

Today sucked! It was one of the worst days so far of this whole damn journey. The CT scan shows that all of William's lymph nodes are swelled with what appears to be active cancer cells. A biopsy tomorrow should confirm this. There is still active cancer in his bone marrow as well. His diagnosis has changed. He has Acute Lymphoblastic Leukemia of the T-cell lineage and Lymphoma and it is also extremely resistant to treatment. He has a very difficult cancer. It appears the Red Devil has the greatest impact on his cancer so it may be that he has to fight the devil in every round now. It will also be critical to go to transplant as soon as he gets to remission because this cancer will keep coming back.

I asked his doctor if William was still treatable and he just looked down at the floor and shook his head. He said, "I told you in the beginning we can't save everyone. I just don't know, his cancer is so aggressive. But we are sure going to try!" The only good piece of news that I can take away from today is that his cancer went from 84% in his bone marrow down to 2%. That's it! That's the best "happy" I can give you right now. And I am not happy, I am pissed, and I am scared. And William, how did he handle the news? At first, not so good, but he called Kaitlyn and talked to her, looked for any silver lining possible, realized this is totally out of his hands and he can't fix it, and then found a guitar...in the hospital...and started playing.

After he had a little time to let it all sink in, we went to the cafeteria to grab a bite to eat while waiting for his room to be ready. He ordered a double bacon cheeseburger, onion rings and a dessert. I mentioned to him I was surprised at how much he ordered (since he has barely eaten anything in the last few months) and he responded, "Well, I might as well eat what I want, it won't be the cholesterol that kills me!"

> *Comment 1: I am so sorry, Amy. I just don't know how my mama heart could take such news. William and your whole family are in my prayers for complete healing and peace throughout this storm. God is mighty!*

> *Comment 9: Amy ...... so sorry ..... I don't know what to say. Nothing I say will make a difference but just know you are not alone. Good things happen when you least expect them ...... my thoughts are with you and all my prayers are for William !!!!!*

> *Comment 20: I am so sorry. We are continuing to surround y'all with love, support & prayers! This battle is not over & with Williams fight and knowing we have a God who heals I'm still standing on that my friend!! Hugs*

Comment 49: My prayers are surely with William and you. I can share good hope, as my son, John, battled leukemia (ALL) 30 years ago, when he was 15 years old. He is now married and his dear wife and he are expecting their first child! Hang on, and pray, pray and pray! God will get you through this!!!! All my love to you and William

August 20

A biopsy on a lymph node in William's neck was done today, and tomorrow he will do the PET scan. The PET scan will help them better pinpoint where the active cancer cells are, if I understand it correctly. They are doing a full body scan so it should be the last piece of the puzzle. His doctor has decided to wait to start chemo until we get these results. They will have a better picture of what is going on and can calculate a chemo cocktail to best go after his cancer. William might get radiation too, but that will only be determined after the results are in. For now, we rest and wait. Right now William is enjoying dinner and a movie from his hospital bed. The hospital experience here at MDA is great and that has helped lift his spirits after yesterday. He is being well cared for here, both physically and emotionally. And we haven't given up hope for good news tomorrow from these new tests.

August 21

The PET scan was done today and now we wait. The doctors put chemo on hold until they get the results from the biopsy and the scan. Then they will customize the right chemo cocktail and get started. We are still hoping for better news than what we heard on Monday, but regardless of what we hear we will move forward with an expectation of complete healing and restoration.

I met several people over the last few days that have been through the stem cell transplant. One person I met was alive today thanks to a double cord transplant. The umbilical cord is a very rich source of stem cells that can be harvested and used for transplants. Most people don't bank the cord due to cost. If the cord is not designated to be banked or donated it is thrown in the trash along with all those life saving stem cells! If you are pregnant or know someone who is, talk about donating the cord. All ladies, talk to your OB/GYN about educating their patients in cord donations. What a beautiful gift as a mom; you give not only the gift of life to your baby, but also the gift of a second chance at life to another. You can learn more about, and sign up for cord donation at www.bethematch.org. Just click on Get Involved and then Cord Blood Donation.

August 22

We have our news. It is both good and bad, but more good. The PET scan shows active cancer in all his lymph nodes (every single one of them) and confirms the chemo just isn't working. That's the bad news. The good news is that they are going to try to get William on one of two clinical trials that have had excellent results in getting resistant patients to remission. They are also going to bring a couple of T-cell ALL specialists in to confer with on William's case. They are not going to administer chemo right now because it just wears his body down and has no effect on the cancer, but it will take a few days to work out all the details so we get to go home for now and have to be back on Monday next week. In the meantime his expanded team will work together to get a new plan for treatment. That's all the technical stuff, here's the bottom line: I asked the doctor if this is treatable, and he said he believes with the clinical trials, yes it is! William will still need the transplant but we have to get to remission first, and hopefully we are on the right path now.

> *Comment 15: You are doing an amazing job with all of this!!! Has he had the chemo nelarabine yet? For us that was the chemo that got Alex into remission. He also had t-cell and the chemo's didn't work he failed induction therapy. Praying for you guys!*

August 23

Dr. Alvarado called me this afternoon to give me an update. I really like that doctor. He said William needs to be back Monday and will be admitted again. They are going to start one of the trial drugs mixed with chemo. His cancer is very aggressive and fast growing, so the hope is that the combo of the drug and chemo will attack it. If this regimen doesn't work they still have Plan B. I still freak out when I hear "aggressive and fast growing," but I have no choice but to trust the doctors and hope in the Lord.

For now, he is enjoying a weekend visiting with his friends. William has been blessed with some pretty amazing friends, and it always lifts his spirits when he gets to hang out with them. I am glad they are there for him.

August 24

We had a nice quiet day today. William upgraded his phone so he has a new toy to tinker with while he is in the hospital next week. I can't wait to see how the clinical trials work, I am hoping for great results (and minimal side effects). William is hoping to avoid the Red Devil, I hope so for him.

August 25

Start sending those prayers for safe travel again. This week Grandpa is going with William. My little ones are having the "Missing Mommy Meltdowns" so this week I am going to stay at home with them. Daddy and William are heading out first thing in the morning, and he will be admitted for the first round of clinical trials with chemo tomorrow. I need all the prayer warriors down on your knees. We *need* these trials to work.

August 26

Dad sent me an update; they have just gotten settled into William's hospital room. He will be there for a couple weeks on this trip. They have decided not to do the clinical trial yet, there are some FDA approved medicines they want to try first. That's even better news because it means we still have a lot of treatment options left. He will be inpatient for about a week and then outpatient for another week while they monitor side effects. Everything can change depending on how he reacts to the medications, but that's the plan right now. They will start chemo tonight; right after he gets some fluids and antibiotics. Here we go!

August 27

The battle with the Red Devil has begun. They started it

last night and unfortunately will repeat it every seven days for 28 days. So William will go four rounds with the devil, plus all of the other chemos that are thrown in the mix. The treatment is very aggressive and to put it in perspective, before, his chemo rounds lasted one week now they will last four weeks. The doctors feel good that this treatment will attack his cancer and get good results. If not, there are other treatment options to try. He is very tired today, and just doesn't feel good, but that's to be expected. Please keep him in your prayers for mild side effects and great results from the treatment and that a match is found soon.

August 28

William slept for about thirty hours, only waking up a few times for short periods. He woke up and is acting more like himself. Sometimes the chemo does that to him, but I am glad he is up and eating finally. He has barely eaten since Monday (two days). Apparently they are talking about discharging him tomorrow and if that is the case, he wants to come home. He will be back for treatment again on Monday but it will be outpatient. We are going to work with MDA and Baylor Dallas to do some of his outpatient care here at home to lessen the travel. The four-hour car rides are very hard on him, especially after chemo treatments. William likes the idea of being at home more.

August 29

William received a new chemo this morning, Pegaspargase (PEG) and seems to be tolerating it alright. He was discharged later in the day so instead of driving late at night, he and Dad are staying the night in Houston then heading home in the morning. He has to be back next week for round two with the Red Devil. We are hoping his blood counts hold over the long weekend and we don't end up in the ER. He hasn't had a transfusion yet with this round of chemo and my fear is when his counts start dropping that they will bottom out fast. We will just have to watch very closely for fever and other symptoms.

September is just a couple of days away, and did you know that September is both National Leukemia Awareness and Childhood Cancer Awareness month; and that orange is the color for leukemia? So do me a favor, during the month of September, everyone rock orange for William and others who are fighting leukemia, for those who have beat it, and for those who lost the battle. Orange ribbons, an orange bracelet, just wear something orange. Then do one more thing, make a personal goal to recruit one person in September to join the bone marrow registry. Most people don't join because they don't know about it. But you can be the voice of hope for thousands who are waiting on their match.

August 30

William and Dad got home this afternoon and he seems to be doing fairly well. The lymph nodes in his neck do not seem as swollen as they were on Monday, before the chemo started. I hope that is a sign that it will be effective and he will go into remission soon. Keep the prayers coming for the chemo to be effective, a 10/10 match to be found soon and for a quiet weekend. He has not had a blood or platelet transfusion with this round of chemo and I worry about his numbers holding for the long weekend. We will be back in Houston next week. I think "On the Road Again" is going to become our theme song.

September 2

We are here in Houston, finally. The traffic here is awful, and it doesn't matter what time of day, it's just always awful. While driving around this afternoon, seeing what's around the hospital, William said he feels like an old car. I asked him what he meant and he said, "Well I am always getting my fluids checked, I am constantly in the shop and I am about to get a new transmission." Just can't argue logic like that. So tomorrow he gets his fluids checked and then has another round of chemo, the Red Devil of course.

September 4

We are back at home for a few days. William had an eleven hour day at the hospital yesterday. But he has decided he likes outpatient chemo versus being admitted for several days. He got his second round of the Red Devil and said it feels like his chest and lymph nodes are on fire inside him. They warned us his blood counts will start dropping pretty quickly over the next several days so we are back on fever watch. But for now he is just happy to be home.

September 5

Today was a hard day. William is not sleeping at night so he is exhausted during the day. He has severe heartburn, hot flashes, nausea, nose bleeds - it just goes on and on. It is so hard to see him this miserable. We met with the doctor at Baylor and are now set up with them for his second lab check each week. William's counts are beginning to drop and with the weekly chemo treatments, his doctor expects them to remain low for several weeks. It is going to be a rough few weeks ahead, but we are gearing up for it. It is really nice to have a local doctor to go to for labs and transfusions. It is great for William too; those four-hour car rides are hard on him.

There are days I just struggle with the fact this is happening to him. It makes it harder when you realize how aggressive his cancer is, and see him so miserable. I still just get mad sometimes, not at God, not at any one person, but at the situation. It's just hard to accept, that's all. I want him to be happy and healthy and vibrant again and I know that's all he wants too. I can't wait for that day.

> *Comment 3: Praying for you - for strength, courage, peace of mind, your own health... I have walked this road (with my husband, not my son - that, I cannot imagine) and I know how hard it is. Hang in there!*

> *Comment 5: Oh Amy....! That day is coming, where William will feel so good! He is strong spirited...just like his "Momma," determined, challenged, and brave! You keep all those too! We love u & love William! Hugs for Alain, James, & Abbey.*

September 7

William's little brother has a stomach virus right now. We have to keep him isolated from William to avoid spreading germs. None of us can afford to be sick right now because we don't want to expose William to any kind of illness. So we need to bathe the whole family (both my parents household and mine) in prayers of healing and protection.

As for William, he said the new antacid is helping quite a bit. He said his bones ache and feel brittle, in his legs especially, so he is going to talk to the doctor about that on

Monday just to be sure it's a "normal" side effect of either the cancer or the chemo. Other than that, he is tolerating the other side effects alright. So far he hasn't had a drastic drop in the blood counts so no ER visits. Let's pray the blood counts hold out till Monday and that this virus doesn't affect anyone else in the family. I can see now that flu season is going to make me a nervous wreck.

September 8

All the prayers worked! James is back to normal today, fever gone and no more throwing up, and no one else has gotten sick. William and I are heading back to Houston very early in the morning. He sees his leukemia doctor and then more chemo. I am not sure when they are going to run the tests to see if this cycle is working but it will probably be towards the end of the month. We are still hoping for a good report with the doctor. Just looking at his neck, the lymph nodes appear to be smaller, so that must be a good sign. The impatient part of me wants to know *now*, but I know that isn't how this works.

September is moving right along, and I have to ask if anyone has taken my challenge to add one more person to the bone marrow registry. For a leukemia patient like William, a stem cell (bone marrow) transplant is his only chance of survival.

Let me just be as blunt as I can be...without the transplant he will die! There are no other options, trust me I have asked. Imagine if you heard those words for your own child. What would you do? You can protect your kids from a lot of things, but you cannot protect them from this. Leukemia hits any one, at any age, at any time. Just a little over three months ago, my biggest decisions in life were "should I do my grocery shopping on Thursday or Friday, and what kind of car am I going to get when my lease is up on this one." Today my life is very different. Every day I think about William and the tens of thousands of people like him that need a match. Every one of those people *belong* to someone. They are someone's son, or daughter, or mom or dad, wife or husband. Every person whom you and I help add to the registry gives these people new hope. I know some people have medical issues that prevent them from joining, but you know people. Talk to the people you know about joining. Do something today to give someone else a tomorrow. Please visit www.deletebloodcancer.org.

September 9

Great news today--great news! We saw Dr. Alvarado, William's leukemia doctor and the minute he walked in the room he took one look at William and said "I have already seen what I needed to." The lymph nodes in his neck are significantly smaller, which means this current chemo cocktail is working! Dr. Alvarado said these are exactly the results he was hoping for. Two more chemo treatments left in this cycle and then they will run the PET scan again to see how much active cancer is left and we will go from there. Overall, it has just been a great day, and I am one happy mama right now!

Flu season is almost here. If you plan to visit William any time during the flu season you will need to get a flu shot before coming over. It is very important that you get the actual injection, not the nasal mist. The mist has a live virus in it. William is not able to get the shot himself and with his compromised immune system we need to help protect him. Thanks for understanding.

September 10

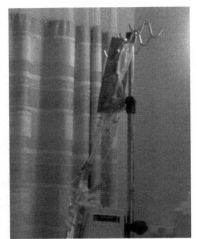

This is the infamous Red Devil chemo. They even put it in a red bag so it looks more ominous. I have mixed emotions about this bag. On one hand it hurts William so much and has a list of side effects that just make you sick thinking about, but on the other hand it seems to be the most effective chemo at killing his cancer. It's a love/hate relationship.

For now, we are back at home after a *long* day. The four-hour car rides are tough on William, especially right after a chemo treatment, but he toughs it out because he just wants to get home. Luckily we will be home for several days before having to head back.

September 11

This round of chemo is taking a toll on William. Progressively through the day the pain in his knees has gotten worse and is pretty much topped his pain threshold. I spoke with his doctor and he said to ramp up his pain meds for a few days to help him. It's one of the side effects of the chemo combo he is on. Please pray for increased strength for him and for the pain to pass. I can't even begin to put in words how much I hate this cancer and what it has done to William. It is profoundly painful to sit helplessly and watch someone you love suffer so much. I hate it, I just hate it!

September 13

If there was ever a time to pray for divine intervention, this is it. William is getting his butt kicked with this round of chemo. He is the weakest I have ever seen him. He told me he doesn't "feel right." I have a call to his doctor and I am beyond worried that he has to endure another round of this Red Devil in just four more days. I am going to ask if they can admit him for it because I truly do not think he has the strength left in him to fight it.

For the time being, I need to request that no one come to visit him. He just isn't strong enough right now. The best way to help now is to pray for him (and get your flu shot).

September 14

There's not much to update today. William is about the same. Not much improvement. I did talk with his doctor and he will evaluate William before they administer the next round of chemo. We can discuss our concerns and determine if admitting him would be in his best interest. Just keep on praying (and I know you are). It's such a hard chemo - and so much of it!

September 15

I am very happy and relieved to report that William has had a better day. He is a bit stronger and feeling better too. All I can say is a very honest and humble "thank you God!" Please pray his match comes soon so he doesn't have to keep taking this chemo.

September 16

We saw Dr. Alvarado today. The incredible swelling in his feet and legs is from one of the chemos, Vincristine. His ankles are the size of my thighs. He is losing feeling in his feet so he is confined to his wheelchair. The doctor feels it is best to stop the last dose of the offending chemo. So tomorrow he will only get the Red Devil. The doctor warned us that some rough days are ahead so we are gearing up for that. It looks like he will stay on weekly chemo for two months, (unless we find a match) but tomorrow will be his last dose of the Red Devil for a while.

September 17

We are home safely. We were stopped on I-45 for over an hour due to a terrible wreck. Several ambulances and two Care Flight helicopters were brought in. We are just really glad we weren't involved in it and sure hope those who were will be okay.

William is tired from the ride, sore from his swelling, and nauseated from his chemo but otherwise in good spirits. I have to hand it to him, he has an amazing attitude. We know some rough days are just around the corner, but he knows they're coming and that they're normal and most importantly, that they will pass. Next week they will run his tests again to see how effective this chemo cycle has been and determine the next cycle. For now, a good night's sleep and a restful day tomorrow are in order.

September 18

William and I would like to ask a favor, a "pay it forward' favor. We are "residents" of the Ronald McDonald House in Houston. This is an amazing place that does so much good for thousands of families with children under twenty-one who are being treated at one of the local hospitals. They provide a home away from home for families who have to travel for medical treatment, at a fraction of the cost of a hotel. They also have eight kitchens where families can prepare food, to help further reduce the cost of traveling. They are staffed by volunteers, who devote themselves to the needs of their resident families. They are just amazing. But they need some serious help in updating their kitchen tools. All they have are worn-out, old, hand-me-down spoons, spatulas, etc.

I pulled out my Pampered Chef catalog and made a list of the basic tools every kitchen needs (that are dishwasher safe), and I would like to order eight sets so that we can replace what they do have with high quality tools that will last. If you would consider donating any amount of money to help us, we would appreciate it. Just send me a message with your contact info and I will get in touch with you. I am not able to give a tax-donation form, nor am I going to ask for one for myself. I will get a card and sign it with the names of everyone who helps, and then deliver the products when they arrive. It's a small way for us to help and give back to those who have helped us, and at the same time, help the families who have to be there too.

September 19

William is having a better day. The awful swelling in his feet and legs is beginning to subside, and even though he still can't feel his feet very well, he is able to get out of the wheelchair and very carefully walk short distances. Hey, a small victory is still a victory! He is also super excited at how many responses we have received for the "pay it forward" to help the Ronald McDonald House. It's just going to be awesome.

My sister asked me to post this, I copied and pasted so these are her words:

"Hi I am William's Aunt Kelly. I asked Amy if I could hijack one of her posts and here I am. Due to a physical disability I am not able to give blood or register on the Bone Marrow registry. I have been wracking my brain as to what I can do to help William or someone else in his situation. I am growing my hair out to donate it; all you need is a 6 – 8 inch pony tail. The other thing to think about is that we are nearing the end of the year and most companies will be having annual enrollment for insurance. To gear up for annual enrollment a lot of companies will also host a health fair or blood drive. If your company holds this type of event, talk to your HR department and see if they would include a blood drive or a swab party. All you have to do is ask. The worst that could happen is that they will say no, the best is someone at your company could save a life.

Amy Roseman at Delete Blood Cancer can help set it up. You could also contact someone at Be the Match to help. Sorry I don't have a contact with them. Carter or Red Cross can help with blood drives. Doing these in Williams name is awesome. However some companies won't or can't host one for an individual. Why not host one for awareness of all blood cancers. The more people we get on the registry, the more lives we can SAVE. The life we save could be William's, your nephew, or maybe even yours. You just never know what God has planned."

September 20

This last round with the Red Devil was not as bad, maybe because William only had the one chemo, instead of the two. The swelling is getting better too. Next week William will undergo the PET scan and bone marrow biopsy to determine how successful this cycle of chemo has been. He gets one last dose of chemo in his spinal column to finish out the cycle. This sounds scary, I know, but it is critical to protect his brain. After the results come back and we know the success rate, Dr. Alvarado (his leukemia doctor) will set a date for the next cycle of chemo to begin. This will be an eight week cycle, but the Red Devil is not in this round, just a bunch of other ones.

I just hope and pray a match is found soon so he can get the stem cell transplant and get off this horrible chemo. Trust me; this is not a long term solution. Keep talking to people about joining the registry, and please consider asking your HR person to include a blood drive and a bone marrow drive when they do open enrollment or health fairs. Kelly had a great idea. It honestly does save lives.

We heard just last week of a man who has waited for two years for a match. Having to be on chemo for two years, can you even imagine? He got his match last week and is getting ready for his transplant in three weeks. Sadly though, too many die waiting on a match because their bodies just can no longer withstand the chemo. I know in my heart, William's match is out there, and I know it will happen in God's timing. But the waiting is awful. When you know your child's life hangs in the balance, it is very hard to wait.

September 23

We are back in Houston for a few days. Tomorrow will be a very long, grueling day. William will have a bone marrow biopsy, PET scan, followed by a spinal tap with a dose of chemo into his spinal column. The day starts at 6:00 a.m. with blood tests, and we don't know how long all this will take. We are just praying for strength and great tests results. We should know the results by Thursday as to how effective this last round of chemo was. From there, his doctor will determine how to move forward. I am nervous and excited.

After we got settled in at the Ronald McDonald House, Dad and I went downstairs to put some ice packs in the freezer and met Dodie Osteen, Joel Osteen's mom. She said the most beautiful prayer for William; it just gave me goose bumps. She visits the hospitals and Ronald McDonald House to visit with, and pray with the families. William missed meeting her as he was resting after the long drive. He is tired and not looking forward to tomorrow, but otherwise in good spirits. And he was able to walk a little more today and said it felt good to get out of the wheelchair for a little bit.

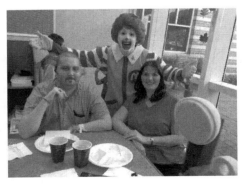

September 25

Today was just plain fun. William had a long day of testing yesterday, but today he had a break from appointments so we drove around and found some neat places. We discovered a fabulous little establishment called The House of Pies, a whole section of antique shops, the local Costco and the Museum of Natural Science. We finished the day by having dinner with Ronald McDonald.

September 27

There's no place like home. We are back and settling in. I had internet trouble on this trip so I decided to save the update till we got home. This will be long, but well worth the read.

Tuesday was an 11 hour day of testing and waiting. It was awful for William. I was in the room with him when he got the spinal tap and chemo injected in his spine. Let me just say, that is something a parent should not witness! When it was over he said I was paler than he was. But sitting there and watching him wince and grit his teeth in pain, I was just sick to my stomach when it was over. That night he fell sound asleep before nine o'clock, and I don't think that boy has *ever* been asleep before 9:00 p.m. in his life, even as a small child. He was exhausted though, in his words, "I have had my spine drilled twice, radioactive fluids mainstreamed into my veins, and poison injected into my spine." He was joking, but there is a lot of truth to what he said.

On Thursday we saw his stem cell doctor and his leukemia doctor and they both had great news for us. First Dr. Champlin (his stem cell doctor), said they received a blood sample from a *possible* match! They were testing it in the lab as we were speaking to determine if it was a close enough match. We will know in about a week or so. That was the best news I have heard in a very long time, and now we just wait to hear - wait and pray. Then we saw Dr.

Alvarado and got the results from the bone marrow biopsy, spinal tap and PET scan. All were fabulous! The preliminary results from the bone marrow show only a 1% blast. That's medical terms, in layman's terms; anything under 2% is considered remission. His PET scan was also great; it showed "excellent therapeutic response" to the first cycle of chemo. So in plain English...based on all the test results, WILLIAM IS IN REMISSION! The goal now is to continue the chemo so that he *stays* in remission.

Since his cancer has proven to be aggressive and resistant to treatment, he has to continue weekly treatments to keep his cancer from coming back. The weekly chemo will keep his blood counts low and continue to abuse his immune system, so we still have to keep the same precautions as before. He will take a one week break from chemo right now because his liver has taken some pretty hard abuse during the first cycle and is showing signs of damage so they want to give him a break to rest the liver, then resume. He will continue the weekly chemo until a match is found (hopefully very soon) and he can go to transplant. Since he responded so well to the first cycle, his doctor has approved for him to do the next cycle of chemo closer to home. William is very excited that he will not have to travel so much.

Just a couple of "housekeeping" things I need to address, if you want to visit William be sure to call Aunt Kelly to schedule. His white counts are pretty low right now, which make him susceptible to infections and he had to be taken off some of his antibiotics temporarily to give his liver a break. So he is at risk of infections, more so than before. Be sure to call! Also, if you have not already done so, get your flu shot (the injection, not the nasal mist as it contains a live virus). And last, I am turning in the order for the kitchen equipment for the Ronald McDonald House on Saturday. If you want to contribute, be sure to message me and let me know by Saturday. And a big thank you to those who have already sent your check to help. I will post the final amounts when everything is in.

September 29

Waiting to hear about our possible match is driving me crazy! Every time my phone rings I just pray it's a Houston number. I know the doctor said it would be a week, but it is so hard to wait.

William is glad to have a week off chemo, but his knees and legs are still hurting pretty bad from the last dose on Tuesday. The week off will be good for him to rest and rebuild strength.

October 1

What a day, what a day! It was one of those where so many things go wrong you want to crawl back into bed and start over. We had William's Baylor appointment this morning. On the way in, a raccoon darted out from the ditch and ran right under my car (not a happy ending). I ran into traffic on every highway trying to get there and Dad had a flat tire. It took two hours to get there; needless to say we were late. But some of the nurses were stuck in the same traffic and they were late too, so in the end everything was fine. William's blood work is okay; his numbers are steady declining which is normal and expected from his chemo Tuesday. He will begin the next round of chemo next week, and his doctor at MDA has approved Baylor to administer this next round.

After William's appointment we went and got him a walker (with a seat) so he can get out of the wheelchair and still be safe when his legs give out on him. The cane is great for balancing but it doesn't do anything to prevent him from falling when he loses feeling in his legs. He is enjoying a week off from the chemo. He is not overly excited about starting back up next week, but understands the necessity to keep his cancer from coming back. I broke down and called the Match Search Coordinator to get an update on our pending, hopeful match. I had to leave a message so maybe I will hear back tomorrow.

Altogether we raised $300 for the Ronald McDonald House and with using host credits and commission, that $300 will purchase more than $500 of products for them. That's great! But it gets even better, my former Pampered Chef teammates jumped in to help too and they are bringing items to donate to the team meeting next week. When it's all said and done, I will repost the total dollar value of what we were able to collectively do for this incredible organization. And of course I will post a photo of all the goodies. Thank you to everyone who helped out.

October 2
WE HAVE A MATCH! WE HAVE A MATCH! WE HAVE A MATCH!! THANK YOU GOD, WE HAVE A MATCH!!!

Comment 1: Holy shit that's amazing!!

Comment 5: A million likes!!!!!!!!!!

Comment 11: Like Like Like Like Like Like Like Like Like!!!!! Praise God!

Comment 20: Fantastic news! Tears of joy for you! God is Good!

Comment 27: Amen and PTL....I am so happy Amy words cannot fully express my heart! WILLIAM know u are prayed for by all of us at Grace Baptist Church

Comment 35: Thank you so much for much for this we just thank you Lord for answering the many prayers and keeping your arms around the family when all seemed lost...

Comment 43: Amy my love, I am bawling and my arm hairs are standing on end. Praise God from whom all blessings flow. Love you!

October 3

I cried all day yesterday, but very happy tears! I can't even adequately express how happy we are right now. So many parents never get to make that post; so many families have to bury their loved ones before a match is found. I spoke with the Search Coordinator again today and she said William's match proved to be much more difficult than originally thought. This match is a miracle! I don't want anyone to think that this is just a "lucky break." This was the hand of God moving to answer the prayers of His faithful! All of your prayers made a difference and we are so grateful to you for faithfully lifting William up.

His match is a 9 out of 10 match, but Dr. Champlin said the one area where it is a mismatch is the least important area; in fact if he could choose one area to have a mismatch this would be his choice. He said this is a near perfect match and he wants to move toward transplant. It looks like it will be happening in about four to five weeks. This time frame could change at any time depending on when the donor is ready, but this gives us a reference for now.

In the meantime, chemo resumes next week to keep his cancer from returning. Keep praying for a successful transplant and for all the financial issues to run smoothly and seamlessly. Also, pray for his donor. What a wonderful gift this person is giving and there is no possible way to thank or repay him or her.

October 5

I have spent the last several days thinking back. It has been nearly four months since we heard those words, "your son has leukemia." At that time I had no idea what to do. I was in a stupor for weeks, I kept waiting to wake up and find out it was just a horrible nightmare. I cried myself to sleep every night for over a month. I just wanted my son back, I just wanted him healthy and whole again and I begged God not to take him from me.

Six weeks ago we were given a very grave diagnosis, and we walked forward knowing that William's only hope for survival was this transplant. William and I were alone on that trip and we talked on the way home. We discussed the hard reality of what he faced and talked about the "what if's." We talked about what to do if the worst happened. But William also told me this; he said "I know without the transplant there is no hope, so this is my only option. If it works, I get to live. If it doesn't, I will die but I get to go to Heaven. So really I am a winner either way!" That was one of the most peaceful moments of this whole ordeal. To know he was at peace, even though he was still a little scared.

Now here we are. God provided him a match and now we wait to hear a transplant date. William is both excited and scared. I think the whole family is. Now we just have to keep trusting through the next steps. Keep praying and keep trusting. The road ahead is hard and long but with your continued prayers I believe William will come out of this healthier and stronger than ever before.

October 7

William starts round two of this chemo cycle tomorrow. This round will include Vincristine, this is the one that put him in the wheelchair, so please keep him in your prayers. Dr. Alvarado cut the dose in half in hopes of minimizing the side effects, but he will have a few new chemos in this round too, and we don't know how he will respond until it happens. I am a nervous wreck right now. I know the chemo is critical in keeping the cancer away but I always worry about side effects, blood counts – everything.

He will continue this cycle until we check in at MD Anderson for his transplant. We check in with his leukemia doctor next week and hope to have a transplant date by then. I can't believe we are so close.

October 8

Today was a challenge for William. He had a six hour chemo infusion. My dad took him this morning, and a sweet friend watched my little ones so I could take them some lunch and sit with him for a little while. When I came around the corner and saw William sitting there it was all I could do to fight back tears. I don't really understand that, I mean it has been four months now.

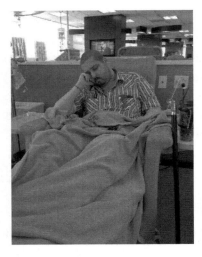

Wouldn't I be used to this by now? But today was one of those days when I just couldn't wrap my heart around this.

I keep reminding myself of all the blessings and how God has remained faithful. Of how He provided a match for William, of how much hope there still is. This transplant, even though there are many unknowns, is still new life for William. I keep thinking of the verse "Look, I am about to do something new; even now it is coming. Do you not see it? Indeed I will make a way in the wilderness, rivers in the desert." (Isaiah 43:19). I have thought about that verse since I heard that William's blood type will change after his transplant and he will adopt his donor's blood type. This is amazing to me, that his very blood will change and be new. New and cancer free! Yes, even on the hard days there is much to be thankful for and there is still hope!

Comment 2: Continued prayers and {{hugs}}! I don't think it ever gets "easy" to see. My heart aches for you! Much love!

Comment 4: As one who has not only stood, but also walked in your shoes, I know your feelings oh so well, and your post tonight brought tears to my eyes. The thing is, my friend, I don't think you ever get used to it. You just keep putting one foot in front of the other ... you just keep running, because if you dare to stop, it will all catch up with you.

Wishing you peace tonight.

Comment 6: as Tamara say's Amy it doesn't, my eye's are tearing up just reading what you wrote, I want to also just give William a big hug!! and you as well, I don't understand either, I look also at my beloved Joel, and my heart breaks as well, Jeremiah 29:11 states " For I know the plans I have for you says the Lord, They are plans for good and not for disaster, to give you a future and a hope." my husband on Sunday night was sharing Ephesians 6: 10 where it states "Be Strong in the Lord and in the POWER of His Might" God the Almighty, Lord of Lords and Kings of Kings, He is Everlasting to EverLasting, that is the power we Stand Firm in, Stand Strong in, the Strength, the Faith, in knowing that He is in Control.

October 9

William is still struggling with his chemo side effect. Please keep praying for him. He started four chemos yesterday (Dexamethasone, Cyterabine, Cyclophosphamide and PEG) and they have gotten the best of him. He is nauseated, can't eat and is very weak. This is a very long, hard cycle and will continue until he is admitted for transplant. We are anxiously waiting for that date. His body has been through so much, and he is just worn and tired. He still has two more chemo treatments this week and four back to back days of it next week plus chemo pills for the next twelve days. Vincristine will be added into the mix in two weeks. He will need a lot of prayer and support to get through this.

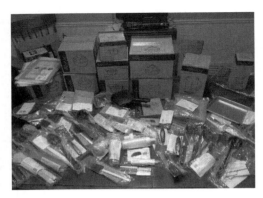

On a different note, I want to give a huge thank you to everyone who donated to the Ronald McDonald House in Houston. We gathered over $700 in products for this amazing organization. I will deliver these products on October 14. There are so many products here, it completely covers my table - and warms my heart.

October 11

I am so glad this week is over. Four days of back to back chemo treatments and three different chemos at one time. William gets to rest this weekend and then he repeats it again next week. His blood counts are borderline but not low enough to require a transfusion, so we are back on fever watch this weekend, as they could drop at any minute and he will need blood. We check in at MD Anderson next week and hopefully will have a transplant date. We are just praying for a transplant date.

October 12

I asked William if he was doing okay today, and for the first time his answer was no. For months he has always answered "I'm okay" even though we know he is miserable. He just doesn't complain. But today he said "No, chemo sucks and I am nauseated all the time!" We see his doctor on Monday in Houston and I am going to ask about some stronger medicine for relief. In the meantime, if you have any ideas or suggestions for chemo nausea relief, please share.

Comment 1: Ginger snap cookies or ginger tea. Ginger helps nausea. Hang in there, William. You've almost got this beat. The finish line is just around the corner and you're going to have an awesome testimony that will change lives. You've got this!! We're all still praying for you!

Comment 5: Has anyone at MD Anderson given you any ABH? They compound it themselves and it comes in a capsule. It works great, but puts you to sleep. When I was having my worst nausea, I was taking it regularly. I was sleeping about 20 hrs a day for a couple of weeks, but I wasn't nauseated. By the way, ABH stands for Ativan, Benadryl and Halidol. No wonder it works so well!

Comment 8:   Phenergan comes in tablet, suppositories, and topical. It helped my momma when she was doing chemo.....good luck

Comment 10: Ginger root, you shred it on a cheese grater and put it in a drink and slam it down. It works wonders. I went through transplant myself 10 months ago and I promise it works. I drank it 7-10 times a day. Praying for William! You got this.

Comment 11:   Ginger and 7-up....or ginger ale. There is also another drink made with ginger in the soda aisle. There is also ginger candy...but I love the pink ginger that comes with sushi. I'm strange like that. Good luck dear!

Comment 12: The cookies I have for him are ginger cookies. I can bring them to you tomorrow. Just need directions to your house. My neighbor makes them and free for cancer patients. He has had so many cards/letters about how much his cookies have helped. Google them @ Doc's oldkinda cookies. Known by many.

Comment 16: I've heard peppermint - like the candies. They did work, to an extent, during pregnancy.

October 13

I have to say, I really appreciate William's leukemia doctor. Dr. Alvarado answered a desperate e-mail on a Sunday afternoon and called in a prescription for Zofran. Now I am just praying for some sweet relief. Thank you for all your suggestions (and cookies). Unfortunately it was getting worse so we hope the new medicine helps him. We leave very early in the morning back to Houston to see Dr. Alvarado. Keep us in your prayers for safe travels. I just don't want William to be miserable for the four hour car ride.

I hate this cancer! I am praying for a day when the cure doesn't involve chemo or a transplant!

October 14

Not the best news today. The results from William's last bone marrow biopsy came back with increased cancer cells. Not terribly increased, but still up. They will recheck after this round of chemo and if the number of cancer cells is still elevated they will make adjustments to his chemo and try a new cocktail to go after it.

Right now we are about to start the blood transfusion and fluids, so we have about another five hours to go.

October 15

We had two back to back eleven hour days at the hospital. We got back to Dallas today and headed to Baylor for William's chemo treatment, and he needed two more units of blood. Mom and Dad came up and relieved me so I could take my two little ones home. It will be a very late night for Mom, Dad and William. Tomorrow we go back for more chemo, including some injected into his spine. Then off to another appointment. I wish I could say he could rest Thursday and Friday, but he has to be back for more chemo on both days and potentially for more blood transfusions since his numbers are dropping again.

I don't say any of that to complain. To be honest, considering the severity of William's cancer, and its aggressive nature I am insanely grateful to still have him with me. I don't mind trekking across Texas for treatments and eleven hour days at the hospital. I just wish it were easier on him. He misses sleeping in his bed when we are away, and he hates staying in the hospital. When we got to MD Anderson yesterday, his heart rate was 145 and his doctor was talking about admitting him and William wanted no part of that. He just wanted to get his blood and go home. Luckily, he didn't have to stay overnight.

For now, we are back home (for a little while), then back to MDA for another bone marrow biopsy. They are going to recheck the number of cancer cells and hopefully they will have gone back down so we can proceed with his transplant. It's going to be a very long wait between now and when we get the results.

October 16

William had chemo today, and will have more on Thursday and Friday, then get to rest for the weekend. I noticed he looks pale and his lips are gray again. After three blood transfusions you would expect him to "pink up" a little, so that's our clue to watch him close. He may need more blood soon. We finally have the nausea under control, with the help of some strong medicines. Now if we could just get him to eat. He doesn't have much of an appetite right now.

His MD Anderson doctor sent me an email today and reminded me that William is in a very serious stage of his treatment and we absolutely must take every precaution possible to keep him safe. Therefore, it is critical that if you plan to see him, you must have your flu shot. Be sure to take the injection, not the nasal mist. If you have a medical reason that prevents you from taking the shot, let his Aunt Kelly know when you call to set a time to visit with him.

I forgot to let you know that William and I delivered the Pampered Chef kitchen tools to the Ronald McDonald House on Monday, and they were thrilled. They had fun going through the boxes and bags and setting everything out in the kitchens. It was like Christmas. They were so thankful. Thank you again to everyone who helped. You may not realize it, but you were a huge blessing to literally thousands of families.

October 18

I am really hoping we don't have to make an unplanned emergency trip to MDA tonight or this weekend. But William isn't doing very well. His white cell count and platelets are extremely low, he has mouth ulcers, and the severe nausea is back. It's like he is unraveling right before my eyes. I have a call into Dr. Alvarado to see if he wants me to bring him in. But every fiber of my "Dr. Mom Radar" is telling me something is WRONG! Once I talk to his doctor I will know more, but for now...prayers...just prayers...lots of prayers!

October 19

I was able to touch base with William's leukemia doctor, and we both agree he needs blood. He does not think it is so critical that I have to get William to Houston right now, and that it will be okay to wait until Monday morning. We are to be back at MD Anderson on Monday for labs, blood and a general check up. I really like Dr. Alvarado. He answers e-mails on nights and weekends for one, but I tease him that he is a control freak when it comes to his patients care. But being a control freak is a good thing in this case. He checks, re-checks and triple checks everything. He looks at all aspects of his patients and will make adjustments to the chemo or medications if he needs to. I totally, completely trust him. He will look at William's labs on Monday and adjust his chemo dose for Tuesday.

He advised us to be on fever watch and keep an eye on his vitals this weekend and to take every precaution we can, as William has no immune system of his own right now. If for any reason we feel he needs to be seen, we are to get him to MDA. So my bag is packed and car is gassed up and ready at a second's notice.

October 20

10:44 p.m. We are back in Houston. William started running a slight fever and having some very minor chest pains. We are at MDA in the ER now. They have run some tests and we are waiting for the results.

11:28 p.m. Well, the nurse just came in and as expected he needs blood, two units actually. The ER doctor said we will be here overnight. We are still waiting on other test results. Thank God we are here; chalk another up to the Mom Radar!

11:58 p.m. He will need four units of blood! Thank God we didn't wait to bring him. In addition to being extremely low on blood, William has double pneumonia. Never saw that coming. No coughing, no symptoms. He is being admitted.

> *Comment 5: Moms know best.*
>
> *Comment 6: Mom's do know best, something God gave us, Doc's should know to listen to Mom's...*
>
> *Comment 10: Thankful for the Mom radar. Praying for you guys!*
>
> *Comment 11: Prayers and great thoughts are with you all. Don't ever doubt a mom's radar it's hooked to her heart.*

October 21

Its 3:00 a.m. I am tired but can't sleep. William is finally asleep and they are about to start his blood transfusions. He will get four units of blood and one of platelets. I don't know how long he will have to stay in the hospital. He hates being here so hopefully not very long.

I am still in shock that all of this is happening to my son. Not just the pneumonia, the whole cancer thing. Cancer isn't supposed to happen to my child. It's just something you see on a St. Jude's commercial, and you think, "Oh wow, that poor child!" But one thing I have learned is that it does happen, and it happens a lot. Every week I hear of another child or young adult dying from leukemia. You can't stop leukemia from happening so what do you do? From experience, I can tell you a few things. First you slow down. When the realization hits you that you might actually lose your child to cancer, you just want to stop time and hold on to every minute, every second! Time loses relevance somewhere along the way.

Then you realize that you have no control of anything. I always considered myself to be an organized and put together person. Always have a Plan B, that's my motto. But cancer has its own agenda and you don't get to give your input. You can't rush treatments; you can't stop chemo side effects. You can't make this go away! When William was a little boy, Mommy's kisses fixed anything, but I can't fix this. There is no pain as great as watching your child suffer and knowing you can't do a damn thing!

But somewhere along the way, you find comfort in the fact that you are not in control. When you realize you can't create a match, or heal him, or save his life, you have no choice but to rely on God. It is the ultimate test of faith, to trust your child to someone else. You can say "I believe, I believe," but when it really gets down to it - WHAT do you believe? Do you believe He can? Do you believe He will, and will you trust...no matter what? I have seen so many miracles happen in the last several months that there is no other explanation for them than that they are from the hand of God. I can't see into the future, but I still have peace at heart. Why? Because I know God loves William even more than I do, and His plan is perfect. My job is to trust that He is who He says He is: All Mighty, Healer, Provider, God of all flesh; nothing is too wonderful for Him.

Another thing that happens is you open your eyes to the world around you. You see the needs of others, not just your own. I heard once that you should be kind to everyone you meet because you don't know what battles they are fighting. That phrase has more meaning to me now. It is so much a part of my life that it has life and breath now. Sometimes you learn that their battle is even greater than yours. So look for ways to be a blessing to others. You have no idea how your random act of kindness will impact another. You may be the only sign of hope they have.

In short, and before my battery dies, call your mom and dad and tell them you love them. Take a day off and just enjoy it with your kids. Read an extra bedtime book. Eat Oreos for breakfast. Life is precious, savor every minute with those you love!

Comment 7: I will be a better person for what I just read.

Comment 9: I am praying for you both. God made a special person when he made you to be William's Mom. You're right it's the hardest thing to let someone else take care of your child, but what better choice than our Lord and Savior.

Comment 12: Amy, have you any idea how much we all love, respect and cherish you? Praying for all of you.

Comment 15: Wow, boy did those words sum it all up!

Comment 18: My dear Amy....you are SO right..cancer is AWFUL....you feel like you have been run over by a semi...but if there was one thing I learned...it was to live and love like there is no tomorrow and to take nothing for granted...going thru this changes your whole life and how you look at tomorrow. The first thing I do every morning is to thank God for allowing me one more day...I have done this for the last 34 years.

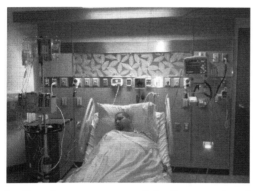

12:22 p.m. Pray now for William. He is reacting to his blood transfusion.

10:28 p.m. William had a reaction to a blood transfusion today. It has happened before but never to this degree. He began to shiver so we added blankets. He was tucked in under five blankets but was still shivering so I grabbed his coat and covered him. Then we grabbed blankets out of the warmer and wrapped his head and feet in warm blankets. His lips turned blue, and his skin was so cold! He began to shake so violently, he was convulsing. I laid on his chest trying to hold him as tight as possible to help control the shaking. He looked at me and through his shaking and convulsing said, "Mama, I'm so cold!" His heart rate climbed until it topped at 160 and even though he was violently shivering and cold, his fever spiked at 102.3.

The nurses and doctor were very urgent in their care but never panicked. I knew it was very serious, but under control. But seeing his reaction and holding him and looking into his eyes during the worst of it was a very surreal moment. You could see how fragile his health is in that moment. The whole episode lasted almost seven hours. Once they were able to get his heart to a stable level, he just fell sound asleep from exhaustion. When he woke up and came to, he didn't know what day it was. More than likely he will not remember most of today. His heart rate is still high, in the 130's but it is down from 160. His fever is slowly coming down too. Still at 100.3 but it's going in the right direction. Dad is staying with him tonight in the hospital room and I am at Ronald McDonald House (supposed to sleeping but that isn't really happening). He still needs blood so they may try to transfuse again tomorrow if his vitals are stable. Thank you for all your prayers. Please keep lifting William up for God's continued healing and mercy!

Comment 1: Oh Amy! I'm so sorry for what he's having to endure. So sorry for your breaking heart. I can't even image the fear you must have felt. I'm praying hard for him and for you.

Comment 4: I know it's easy to say and hard to do but keep your faith. A lot of us have been in William's position. He WILL be himself again soon

Comment 7: Our most gracious Heavenly Father, we thank you for this day and your many blessings we receive every day. We ask to please give William the strength to rest peacefully tonight and help him gain strength to face tomorrow. Please take him in your arms and heal his body, this we ask in Jesus name .... Amen

Comment 8: I cannot imagine everything you and William have gone through, and then this today! My heart breaks. I was reminded of Papa God's words today in a women's bible study from Matthew 11:28-39 where Jesus understands the hurts and aches of the soul and offers true rest in Him. I pray that you and your family can do that tonight...rest in Him.

Comment 14: God gives us strength when we do not think we have an ounce left....William will always feel the love around him even if he doesn't remember the moment. Prayers and more prayers

Comment 16: OMG that happened to Daniela, but after ARA-C chemo. She was shivering so badly, I cover her with my body and hold her tight. Also her BP went down to 70/20 and they transfer her to ICU. Her heart beat was around 150. Scariest time ever. Dr wanted to put her on ventilator and in coma to help her heart. Luckily her BP went up with all the meds they were giving her.

October 22

When William woke up this morning he was alert and his vital signs were stable. He has almost no memory of the last few days. He remembers going to the ER and being moved to the hospital room but it goes foggy from there. He said all he really remembers from yesterday is Dr. Alvarado coming to see him, "a haze and the numbers 102." He didn't know the 102 was his fever. His CT scan showed multiple pneumonia pockets, and as of right now he still needs more blood so they have prepped him for another transfusion. They are starting it right now as I am typing. There is a team of nurses watching him close and will check his vitals every 15 minutes for signs of a reaction. I am very nervous. He is too, after hearing what happened yesterday.

I think something in my mind or my senses has gone into hyper-drive. Everyone has feelings of déjà vu from time to time, but I have been stuck in a constant state of déjà vu since William was stabilized yesterday evening. Maybe it is from seven hours of stress and trauma, I really don't know but it is a very weird sensation. Has anyone ever had that happen to them?

> Comment 1: yes and under stress it is worse...because you are worried and hyper...and probably without good rest...just know we are all praying for him around the clock...and though you are related to him...we pray as if he was our own...diligently....to a much greater power than you, us or the doctors....bask in the knowledge that he is loved and being cared for by streams of angels...doing what is best for him...we love you all...

> Comment 4: I have had that happen. It's because his illness is not easily cured so you are going through the same thing over and over again. I went through that with Sarah for her first 6 months of life when we couldn't get a "working shunt" and she kept having to have surgery. The good news is, it's so overwhelming and traumatizing that I don't remember the details and it seems like a lifetime ago. Your mind can't handle what is going on, you are in shock, it's your mind/body's way of handling all of this. I will never understand why things like this happen to

good people. Just keep praying even when you are weary and tired.

Comment 6: Prayers and faith have helped you through the last few days. Try to continue . You admitted last night that you hadn't even rested and it goes without saying that your under tremendous stress. This doesn't mean that your feelings aren't real. The body try's to protect and heal itself. It's your great instincts that allowed you to tune into getting William help. But you must take care of yourself to care for William. Prayers are with you all. Now that the nurses are aware of the previous problem they will be a step ahead.

October 23

Today William will receive one more unit of platelets (if they are available) and one more unit of blood. His blood pressure has remained a little high after yesterday's transfusion so they are trying to control that with medicine. After his transfusions they will administer his chemo. He is a day late in getting his chemo and with his cancer cells on the rise in his last bone marrow test, his doctor did not want to hold off any longer with the chemo. We just can't let his cancer get a foot-hold here. They are increasing the pre-transfusion medications with the hope of stopping any reactions. It's a little nerve wracking but there aren't any other options. He has to have the blood, and he has to have the chemo.

I have noticed a common thread between the different hospitals that have treated William, and that is a shortage of platelets. They are running short here at MDA too.

Surgery patients get them first, and then what is left over is given to patients based on need. Some patients, who need them, won't get them! Donating platelets takes a little longer than donating blood, about two hours. Please, if you can, go donate platelets. Patients like William need them.

October 24

Here's a staggering fact; MD Anderson goes through 650 units of blood a day. William's nurse said that leukemia patients in particular use more blood products than other cancer patients because they lose more hemoglobin and platelets than others. Also the chemo used for blood cancers are the harshest ones with worse side effects. I am asking again, if you are able to donate blood or platelets please do. The need is great. I have donated blood many times, but I donated platelets this morning for the first time. It takes about two hours but you can donate more often, and you do honestly save lives. My sweet friend Denise came and donated with me.

William is improving now. He has received four units of blood, two units of platelets and one immune globulin, plus he gets breathing treatments every six hours and nonstop antibiotics. His vital sign are in the normal range now and he really wants to go home. We are hoping very soon. He has had about as much fun and excitement as he can stand. Plus the fact his 21st birthday is next week and he doesn't want to spend it in the hospital!

October 25

Oh, my chest just aches with every beat of my heart! Maybe it's the calm after the storm but it does. I guess I am wearing my grief and worry. A man stopped me and took my arm and said to me "It's okay, God can handle this." He didn't even know what "this" is but he could see the struggle within me just by looking at me.

William was discharged this evening but we have to stay close to MDA and be back on Monday morning. He still has a bad pneumonia infection so we have to give him IV antibiotics for a while. They are sending a home health nurse to the Ronald McDonald House to help us with that. Right now, it looks like we will make it home before his birthday.

Meanwhile, back home, my little girl isn't feeling too well and I hate that I can't be there with her, even though I know she is in good hands with her Gammy. It is so hard to be away from my little ones. I am so torn! When I am with William I feel guilty for leaving them, and when I am with them I feel guilty for leaving William.

October 27

The effects of the Vincristine are starting to creep up on William. It's one of the chemos I hate; it put him in the wheelchair. His feet and ankles are starting to swell and the bone pain in his legs is getting worse. His inpatient doctor is trying him on vitamin B6 and L-glutamine to see if they help with the side effects. It's part of a study, and I think so far it has helped. It hasn't eliminated the side effects but they are less severe this round than last. He gets another dose of Vincristine on Tuesday and that will be the true test.

We are trying to avoid giving him one of his pain killers as it has a very serious drug interaction with one of his antibiotics. He only has to take that antibiotic till Friday, so if he can hold out on just the every four to six hour break-through pain meds till then, we can avoid a potentially fatal issue. It only happens in less than 1% of cases, but seriously, who is willing to risk that you might be one of the unlucky few?

He still gets his IV antibiotics along with the sixteen other medications he is taking. I am getting used to doing the IV now and it doesn't freak me out as bad as it did. We check his temp and vitals several times a day and record everything. This is just one of the many "faces" of cancer.

October 28

We saw the stem cell doctor today, and William's transplant hinges on the results from the bone marrow aspiration taken today. If the cancer cells are only residual, we will move forward to transplant ASAP. If there are still cancer cells (like the last BMA showed), then they will change chemos and do another round. If the transplant is done while he still has active cancer cells it will increase his chance of a relapse. We will find out the results on November 4. I ask, beg, and plead for everyone to pray for nothing more than residual cells! It will be a long week while we wait for results.

On a happier note, William will be home to celebrate his birthday. I know a lot of his friends read these posts, so I need to speak direct with y'all for a minute. William is super excited to see all his friends but keep in mind he does still have a very serious and active pneumonia infection in both lungs. He is still sick! His white blood counts are also very low, leaving him open to catching anything and everything. We need to avoid crowds of people coming at the same time so please call his Aunt Kelly to arrange a time to visit on Thursday. Also flu shots are mandatory, period - no exceptions. And we will have everyone wear a protective mask and gloves, again no exceptions. I want as many of his friends as possible to come see him, because let's be honest this is not a fun way to spend your 21st birthday. But his safety is my utmost priority and I have no problems turning "Mama Bear" on anyone. It ain't pretty, so let's not go there! I know you guys only want the best for William too, and I appreciate you all helping us keep him healthy as possible.

October 30

We got home late last night. There really is no place like home. William handled the four hour car ride pretty well, and the L-Glutamine is helping with the swelling in his feet and ankles. Tomorrow is William's birthday, and I have much to do. I have to get busy baking and decorating his cake.

October 31

Today is William's birthday! Most of you don't know, but he was a miracle baby. He was not supposed to make it full term, and my doctor tried to terminate the pregnancy to save my life. But what he didn't realize was that baby WAS my life! So with his reluctant approval, we carried on. William was a fighter even before he was born, and he beat the odds 21 years ago. I have no doubts that as he fights again, he will beat the odds with cancer too!

Please take a minute today to wish William a Happy Birthday. Post it here or send him an e-mail to hope4william@gmail.com. Let's show him he is not fighting this battle alone.

Comment 4: *Happy birthday William, You have so much on your plate but, you are a fighter and you will fight through this. Have an amazing day.*

Comment 9: *Happy 21st Birthday, William. Praying you have a good day. Know that I am praying for you as you fight the 2nd battle of your life. Hang in there!*

Comment 15: *William!!! Happy Birthday to one of the bravest guys I am blessed to know!!! Hoping you have a great day today!!!*

Comment 24: *Happy Birthday William, while I don't know you I can tell by your story that God's hand is all over it. God doesn't make mistakes, he has a plan for you and there is a purpose for everything that happens in your life. God is always with you, trust him and have faith! God Bless you always!*

Comment 53: *William, It being your birthday is a mere coincidence of time. Your ability, willingness, strength, desire to overcome such obstacles, certainly serves your name well. "WILL" you are. Having never known you, you have always been included in my prayers. Happy B-Day to you (Will U Are) and I'm not sure a name has ever identified anyone any better...!!!*

Comment 60: *William, you are a Miracle and we will be praying for you to continue to have a lot more miracles throughout your long wonderful life. God bless you and give you peace during this difficult time.*

November 1

Thank you all so much for the birthday wishes for William yesterday. Between comments, emails and texts there were nearly 200 of them. I tried to read them to him but got choked up and started crying. He can always log on, but I think I will print them out and put them on a poster board or something so he can read them anytime he is feeling down. It always lifts his spirits to know so many are thinking about him and praying for him.

We received another piece of great news today; Leukemia Texas has chosen William for their quarterly grant through their Patient Aid Foundation! He will receive $1000 to go towards medical bills and other medical related expenses.

He had an awesome day yesterday, but it took a toll on him. By early afternoon he couldn't keep his eyes open. He fell sound asleep and was hard to wake up for temperature checks and medicine. His blood numbers took a substantial jump so we didn't have to spray anyone down with Lysol (but we did with his gifts and cards). He ran a slight fever in the early morning hours and we worried about having to take another emergency trip to MDA, but by this morning it stayed in the normal range. So for the remainder of the weekend, we are on fever watch and ready to run to MDA if needed.

My parents are taking him for his doctor visits next week; my little girl broke a tooth so I need to take care of her. It is very difficult not going, especially knowing we will hear the results from the last bone marrow test, and the fact that these results determine if he goes to transplant or suffers another round of chemo. Sorry in advance, Mom and Dad but I am going to pester you to death on Monday with calls and texts!

November 3

Tomorrow (Monday) is going to be a big day. I have to take Abbey to the dentist for her broken tooth so Mom and Dad are taking William to MD Anderson to see his leukemia doctor. We will know tomorrow the results of the bone marrow biopsy taken October 28. Everything hinges on these results! If his cancer cells have increased, we abandon the current chemo regimen and try the next option. If they are nothing more than residual, we move to transplant ASAP. I am nervous in ways I can't even express.

William has been sick since he got pneumonia in mid-May. Then of course the leukemia diagnosis came on June 6. The long term illness and side effects of continuous chemo have taken a very deep toll on him, and to be quite frank, I am worried about him. He will not eat unless forced to. Even then it is barely anything. Even his demeanor has changed. I am just worried! We need good news tomorrow, we really do. Part of the battle is emotional, and he needs an "emotional WIN" tomorrow in a big way! Please pray for safe travels and a great report.

November 4

I have the best news to share with you! I had Mom put me on speakerphone while they met with the doctor (pathetic, I know), but William has NEGATIVE minimal residual disease in both the bone marrow and lymph nodes. So in English, that means he is finally in a full remission! I asked why he is so tired, lethargic and weak and the doctor said it is because his cancer was so aggressive that the only way to kill it was to give William extremely high doses of chemo. His body is exhausted and worn from being poisoned at such high levels. Dr. Alvarado said they are going to let him rest for one week from chemo so he can regain some strength and prepare for transplant.

We have two huge prayers requests right now: 1.) We need insurance approval for the transplant (it was submitted on November 1, and we are waiting on the approval). When William turned 21, his Medicaid switched from tradition to a managed-care Medicaid. Traditional Medicaid had already approved his transplant, but it had to be resubmitted to the managed-care plan. Silly, I know. But that's what we have to do. I don't foresee there being a problem since it was approved already, just a formality I guess.

2.) We need to pray the donor is ready the minute we get the approval from insurance so there is no lag-time. If it takes three to four weeks for transplant, William will have to continue these high levels of chemo, and he really needs the break to recover.

November 6

William had a very good day today. The insurance has requested a couple of pieces of information before they approve the transplant. First they wanted to get a dental clearance and second, he has to talk with a social worker from the hospital to make sure he is emotionally and mentally ready for the procedure. A big thanks to Dental Oncology Professionals for jumping through hoops to squeeze us in on short notice. We now have dental clearance! And the interview is scheduled for Friday. We are getting close. I am so excited! It is beginning to feel real now as everything falls into place. Keep praying for the approval, and for the donor.

William was able to hold down some food today - finally! The break from chemo has been good for him. He has been feeling better and even laughing occasionally. He was able to get out of the wheelchair and walk around a little bit. He is still very wobbly on his feet, but eventually the feeling in his feet and legs (once the chemo is behind him) will come back. I so look forward to the day he is strong again. For now, we celebrate every victory, no matter how big or small! We have much to celebrate, and much to be thankful for.

November 8

William had his call from the social worker today. We need to fill out his advanced directives and get them on file with the hospital. The advanced directives are the medical power of attorney and DNR papers. We have known for several months that we need to fill these out, but you cannot imagine what this feels like! William and I have discussed what to do if the worst happens, but it was just a verbal "what-if" conversation. I guess I just don't like the idea of making it so formal. We will be back in Houston Monday so we will get these filled out, and then wait for the approval. This weekend we are back on fever watch. His counts dropped again, and he is neutropenic so we have to be very careful of infections, colds, etc.

After we meet with his leukemia doctor on Monday we will have a better idea of how soon the transplant will happen after insurance approval. He may have to go through another round of chemo, but with any luck it will be a short one and he will be preparing for transplant very soon.

November 9

Did you know of all the money raised for cancer research, only 4% goes to childhood cancer research? Did you know leukemia is the most common childhood cancer and did you know that adults who survive other forms of cancer are more likely to develop leukemia as well? Seems to me a lot more money needs to be put into finding a cure for leukemia! I firmly believe finding the cure starts with finding the cause, but that's a whole different conversation.

November 10

Tomorrow we will see Dr. Alvarado and find out the game plan for the coming weeks. We would appreciate prayers for safe travels and a quick response from the insurance, please. Once we have approval we can get a firm transplant date. I guess William will resume chemo this week unless Dr. Alvarado decides to be extra generous and give him another week break, but somehow I highly doubt it.

November 12

We are back at home now, after a twenty-hour medical marathon. William was able to sweet talk Dr. Alvarado into giving him one more week off of chemo. His lab results show the last chemo dose is still working so it is safe to allow one more week. William is so far beyond exhausted that if the doctor said William would have to resume chemo this week, I was willing to hold the doctor hostage until he changed his mind! Luckily it didn't come to that.

I do have to admit that yesterday was a bit disappointing. While we were there the Stem Cell doctor called and asked us to come see him immediately. Well, we thought they had received the approval or something great. No, he just wanted to give us an update. Everything has been submitted and now we wait. With Thanksgiving looming around the corner and waiting on the approval and then working out the schedule with the donor, we should plan on another four weeks. With the wait being so long William needs to resume chemo. I know four weeks doesn't seem like a long time BUT IT IS! I hate chemo! I hate what it is doing to William! He doesn't even look the same anymore! I hate the nausea, I hate the pain, I hate seeing him suffer so much. He is so physically and emotionally beaten down right now. Everything about him is weak, even his voice. It just makes me so mad to see him like this! I know there is an end in sight, or at least my head knows it!

There is a disconnect between my head and my heart right now. My head says. "It's only four more weeks, he can do this, he is strong." My heart says, "Are you kidding me, he has to suffer another round? LOOK AT HIM! Don't you see him suffering, how the hell can he make it another round?"

I have to keep reminding myself that William is a fighter and he has a great support system to help him. My parents and my sister are amazing. His friends are amazing too. Kaitlyn, his girlfriend, has been by his side through this entire journey. When she isn't at work, she is with him.
 He is completely surrounded with love and support, but we can only do so much for him. The inner battle belongs to him. There comes a point we are just the cheerleading section. Please pray for him, for the next four weeks especially as he endures another round of chemo, and

please pray that the approval comes quickly and the donor is ready at a second's notice so that maybe this process will not take four more weeks, maybe it will move faster for him. Pray for him to physically and emotionally be strong for what lies ahead. Pray for all of us who love and support him to be able to help him in the best way possible.

Comment 1: As a Mum who has walked this path in the UK with our 23 yr old son your are certainly all in our thoughts and prayers x x x x

Comment 4: It's so hard to be patient and transplant delays are VERY COMMON. Matt's initial target for transplant was early Feb, and then things were "delayed," the first more solid date they gave us was 3/9, then the donor needed another week, so it changed into 3/20 as the target. After transplant chemo started it was delayed one more day - his transplant was at 6:09pm on 3/21. He had a mini-cycle of chemo to keep him in remission while we waited. It's so so tough to wait when you just want the torture to stop as soon as possible. Prayers for you and William and his doctors and the donor - hope they can all get it together!!

November 13

I read once that life is not lived on the mountain tops. Life is lived in the journey. Those "mountain top" experiences are few and far between, and most of life is lived in the day-to-day hills and valleys. Cancer is kind of the same way. The mountain tops are getting good test results or the transplant or surgery or finding your match, but the journey is the day to day stuff. The chemo, the pain, the nausea. Eating three bites of a sandwich then vomiting your guts up and having dry heaves for two hours. Taking over 20 different medications a day. Looking at your pillow and seeing your hair all over it. Wondering if you are going to see your next birthday. Getting a doctor's permission to take a new vitamin because it may have an interaction with one of your pills. Looking at your belongings and deciding who gets what in case you don't make it. Using the term "don't make it" instead of "die." Deciding what kind of funeral arrangements in case you "don't make it." Having someone help lift you off the commode because your legs are too weak to stand. Living with cancer every day is hard. Some days are better than others but it is a hard journey, and it's hard for everyone.

Sometimes when I write these updates it is medical stuff. Sometimes it is something William and I have talked about and sometimes it is nothing more than my raw emotions. Because that is what this journey is all about. It's a physical *and* emotional journey. I try to keep this page as "real" as possible in every way because what you read is what is really happening or what we are really feeling. This is how cancer really affects our lives. Some days I am so mad I just want to scream and cuss and cry out of anger, frustration and fear. Other days I handle it much better. I still don't understand "why" and probably never will.

But understand, even on the days I am at my worst I am still okay, and tomorrow will always bring new hope! Always, because even in my sadness and anger, God is faithful - always!

Yesterday I had a bad day (part from disappointment and part from exhaustion), but I sat with William and we talked. He is very grateful for the extra week break from chemo and he is not looking forward to the next round.

But he will do it, and he will fight through it. I asked him "Do you have enough fight left in you for one more round? The end is in sight. It's four more weeks, hard weeks, but you have an end date!" He said yes, he could do it. He *will* do it and he will get through it. His attitude and strength help me tremendously! He seldom complains. He just perseveres through! He doesn't laugh much and seldom jokes anymore, but he will again. He is amazing, I am so proud of him! I told him I had to run to the store and asked him if he wanted anything before he starts the next round and he asked for some white chocolate truffles. I don't know why this makes me laugh but it does. So I am off today to pick him up some truffles.

Just keep on praying, and I know you are, for the days ahead. Keep praying for quick approval and for the donor to be healthy and ready. Pray for extra strength for William and for us as we take care of him.

Thank you for taking this journey with us, for your support, encouraging words and constant prayers!

> *Comment 2: this just made me cry. It will give you the best feeling in the world to get him some truffles because you know they are what he wants. And with so little control, it's those little tiny things that make all the difference.*
>
> *Comment 24: Amy, thanks for keeping it real!*

November 14

A couple of days ago I was thinking about a man whom I used to work with, named Robert. Robert was a prayer warrior, a true man of God. And as most Christians do, he had a past. Robert was also an ex-con. One day we were super busy. William was just four years old, and he needed to use the bathroom. I asked Robert if he would take William to the bathroom for me, which he did. A few minutes later I looked up and here comes William and Robert, hand in hand, returning. Robert came back and sat down and we continued working. I starting laughing and said "Hey Robert, do you realize I just trusted my four year old son to an ex-convict?" We both laughed and he said that was the power of Jesus, that we could see past previous mistakes and the different colors of our skin and still love and trust each other, as a brother and sister in Christ.

The other night I was thinking about Robert, and I was wishing I had a way to contact him, to ask him to pray for William. He was one of those people who just seemed to have a direct line to God. Well, my phone rang about thirty minutes ago, and it was Robert on the other end! He found my old business card with my cell phone and felt like he needed to call me. I told him about William and he is also praying for him now. Sometimes God just amazes me! It's incredible how much hope can be in something as simple as a phone call!

William is also having a pretty good day. He is enjoying his white chocolate truffles and the best malted milk balls on the planet. Dr. Alvarado even let him skip out of doing his lab check today since his numbers looked good on Monday. He hasn't had this long of a break from the doctor or hospital in five months. He got out and went to the game store too, so he has a new game to keep him entertained for a little while. All in all, it was a very good day today. I emailed the hospital to see if they had heard anything on the approval. They haven't heard anything back yet. But that's okay, we have an army of people praying, and God showed me today that He is listening and moving, so I know it will happen.

November 16

Y'all say a prayer for William. He has been doing pretty well and feeling better, but he has started running a fever. Mom and Dad were planning on taking him to MDA this week, but if he still has a fever in thirty minutes, they are going to head out tonight and take him to the ER. It's a four hour drive so prayers for safe travels would be very much appreciated, and of course, prayers for William's health too. It's a low fever right now, but it was low when he had pneumonia a couple weeks ago too, so the worry never stops.

November 17

William's fever went down and stayed down. However, Mom and Dad are taking him back to Houston today. He has some symptoms and pains that probably need to be looked at, and it will be best to be close to the Emergency Room in case he spikes another fever. Tomorrow the chemo starts back up and it's an awfully harsh regimen. He needs lots of prayer to get him through the next two weeks, which will be the hardest part of this four week regimen. He is especially nervous about the 14 day chemo pill (it makes him incredibly nauseous and sick) and for the next two weeks he has to take chemo shots in his stomach for four days each week. It hurts! And this chemo, ARA-C, is the one that craters his blood counts. Plus he will also be getting chemo through IV as well. It's just a LOT of chemo in several different forms, sometimes taken simultaneously. He will need the extra prayers for strength to get through!

November 18

Everyone, please right now pray! William's insurance denied the transplant saying it was experimental and not medically necessary. I think I am going to throw up! I have emailed MDA to find out our options but I need every person praying, and everyone you know praying, and everyone they know praying! Without this transplant, my son will die. There are no other options for him. Please pray, please. Pray as if he were your child.

> *Comment 1: Amy UNREAL. UNJUST. SCREWY PEOPLE. WTH!!!!! Got your back, Williams for sure. Love you all!!!! Here comes the prayer team!!!!!!!!!!!!!*

> *Comment 2: Pardon my French, but....what the HELL? Experimental is what you do when it is ABSO-FREAKING-LUTELY medically necessary!*

> *Comment 5: APPEAL IMMEDIATELY!!! HATE insurance companies with a passion... they are only in the business of making money - not paying claims / saving lives! Go to the top... and you should have the support of MDA in your corner. DO NOT give up.... am praying....*

> *Comment 26: Amy, all I can say is Unbelievable!! if he was a drug addict or had an alcohol problem, he would be fully covered!!! I just wrote the President of the USA about this!!!*

> *Comment 42: I'm so sorry and very angry! 24 yrs ago when transplants were just being done I had*

this problem. We went before the insurance board and won. I just can't believe the insurance is still this backwards. I know prayer always helps but this is one of those times when someone needs to scream till you find the person who made this ignorant decision. And then scream some more. Transplants are NOT experimental now. They are proven life saving medical procedures. I'm so sorry that on top of all you all are going thru that this was added. But trust me the idiots that made this decision is most likely not a medical employee. Prayers are with you.

Comment 58: I am not surprised by the denial - keeping fighting with them though, it might be standard for them to deny it until they have all the test results, etc they are looking for - it's such a shame that insurance companies literally do not care about people and what receiving a denial like this will do to a family that is already going through so much. MDA knows what they are doing and I believe they will get it approved, I'm sure it's not the first time they have dealt with this situation. Has William applied for Medicaid yet? I didn't apply for Medicaid until after matt's transplant, but they pretty much pay for anything that my primary insurance doesn't. I don't know how the application process works in TX though. In PA have to be denied Social Security Disability (which makes no sense to be denied!) And then he qualified for Medicaid health insurance. Amy I am praying for William and now for these JERKS that his appeal gets to the right desk and gets approved. He will get his transplant. Be the Match publishes all kinds of resources for help in

this situation as well. But Fox News and the media
- fantastic way to start!!

November 19

It was a very long night, as you can imagine. I was sick to my stomach and fought the urge to vomit all night. A hundred thoughts raced through my head. I talked with William. He said, "I don't understand. Without that approval they basically just sentenced me to death." I kept hearing those words and thinking of any and all options that we can explore. All of this was going on in my head. But as my worry grew, a peace was growing too. I said in the beginning that I believe nothing is too wonderful for the Lord, and I still believe it. He has proven Himself faithful through this entire process and I do not - WILL NOT accept that He is going to let us down now. It will not happen! One way or another, this transplant is going to happen.

I heard from the hospital this morning, and they are sending an appeal. They added a test that the insurance requested and changed the wording so it is crystal clear that this procedure is not in any way "experimental." She told me their staff is working 110% to get this approved.

If for any reason they deny it again I will begin fundraising. One way or another I believe in my heart that this transplant is going to happen. There are 22 million registered donors and ONE suitable match for William. That in itself is a miracle, and God is still in the miracle business. MDA will be submitting the appeal today or tomorrow, just as soon as they get everything together. In the meantime I need to request that you continue to pray for an approval and please, I cannot stress this enough...continue to pray for his donor. Pray with faith! Hebrews chapter 11 says the following: "Now faith is the substance of things hoped for, the evidence of things not seen."

By faith, Abel...
By faith, Enoch...
By faith, Noah...
By faith, Abraham...
By faith, Sarah...
By faith, Isaac...
By faith, Jacob...
By faith, Joseph...
By faith, Moses...

"Therefore we also, since we are surrounded by so great a cloud of witnesses, let us lay aside every weight, and sin which so easily ensnare us, and let us run with endurance the race that is set before us, looking unto Jesus, the author and finisher of our faith, who for the joy that was set before Him endured the cross, despising the shame, and has sat down at the right hand of the throne of God."

Pray with faith! For He is bigger than any obstacle before us!

Comment 3: If you haven't already start a GOFund me account fundraiser. Start now spreading it to collect donations. Ill spread it everywhere too... Inbox me if you need help. Ill help.

Comment 5: You may have already considered this but just an idea....you might start researching to find out if you could get some financial help thru "Chronic Disease Fund" that is in Carrollton. Pho# 877-968-7233 (toll free). If they cannot help you, maybe they can direct you to another Organization that can help you ! Praying for you !

Comment 17: Keep the faith! When I was a social worker in Dallas, the process is to deny, deny, deny! Those that appeal and keep fighting for help will be rewarded for their efforts. That was the sad reality that I experienced.

Comment 29: The Leukemia and Lymphoma Society here in Dallas can help defray costs also. They helped another friend of mine through his battle with Lymphoma

Comment 30: So sorry the insurance people have their heads up their butts!!! Will pray their heads get extracted.

Comment 58: Believing the Most High God for great and mighty things for William.

November 20

So I get a call today, and someone from the insurance wants to speak to William for an assessment for his transplant. She was pretty rude, and had no interest in speaking to me whatsoever (and made it quite clear). They will call him hopefully tomorrow on his cell phone. I personally think they received the appeal from MDA and are looking for some other reason to deny it since they never contacted him on the first request. You know what to do. Pray this through! Pray for divine protection over William as he deals with this. I will be sure to let you know what happens after the call. Share the post so we have as many as possible praying. Mama Bear has sharpened her claws and we are going to fight this all the way to the bitter end!

Comment 38: Amy ~ do you have a medical power of attorney for William? If you do, the insurance company, doctors, etc., will HAVE to talk to you. If you do not, then get one signed by William immediately. Make sure it is on file with the insurance company, doctors, and hospital. So very sorry you're having to deal with this added aggravation.

November 21

William received his "assessment" call, but he said there wasn't much "assessing" to it. He said she was nice (that's a good thing) and asked questions about his height and weight and the name of his attending physician, etc. The call didn't take too long and he said she didn't ask one single question about the actual transplant. I guess, once again we wait.

We will see his stem cell doctor on Monday and I will get an update if they have received a response. If for any chance they deny it again, I am seriously tempted to post their number so everyone can call and raise a little hell with me! LOL

Right now the effects of this round of chemo have already started making him miserable. He has a rash covering his torso, is very sensitive to touch, and feels like his bones are "bruised." He has swelling in his legs and ankles. Dr. Alvarado has us on fever watch again. If he spikes a fever, we will need to make another emergency run to MDA. It is getting time to find a temporary apartment and go ahead and make the move to Houston. William's body is wearing out, and not as able to fight the chemo effects. Dr. Alvarado has mentioned that due to the complications he is having, we need to be within twenty minutes so he can be treated there if anything happens. So next week, we are going to be apartment shopping.

William told me today that he feels a difference when he takes the chemo now. In the beginning, it made him sick, but he felt strong enough to fight it. Now he can feel the chemo killing him, every time he takes it. He said it is different, it's not just that he isn't strong enough to fight the effects anymore, he literally feels himself dying slowly with every dose. I fear we are running out of time.

Thanks for all your support, help and prayers. Together, we are going to see this happen, We HAVE to!

> *Comment 4: I'll call anyone you want me to! We're praying that certain personnel who have inadvertently misplaced their heads within their hind quarters will soon be able to safely remove them and thus be once again able to make sane and rational decisions!*

> *Comment 8: @Eyin... that is PRICELESS... I SO need to remember that - never heard it so eloquently stated!!! Obviously, the "assessment call" was nothing more than an outright stall tactic!!! Those (empty value) questions are irrelevant to the transplant and the approval... and they KNOW who his attending is!!! <Blood is seriously boiling here!> Pretty sure there aren't many degrees of separation between Satan and Insurance Companies!!! ;(*

November 23

I am not a patient person, and waiting on this decision is driving me crazy! I hope beyond hope we have an answer by the time we see William's stem cell doctor on Monday. And by "an answer" I of course mean an approval!

I am also stressed over this weather. Normally I love the winter weather but I don't love driving in it, and we are supposed to have ice tomorrow. I am watching the news and Texas Storm Chasers very closely to determine the best time to leave to get ahead of it. I figure once we are past Corsicana we should be safe, but it takes about an hour to get to that point. I am loading the car up with lots of blankets. The goal for this trip is to find an apartment too. It's getting time to be closer to MDA on a more permanent basis, and lessen the travel to and from. I definitely have lots of prayer requests for this trip, safe travels, temps to stay above freezing, finding the right apartment and to get that freaking approval!

I have some good news to share. I heard through an email that someone learned about, and joined, the bone marrow registry from reading William's page and they are a match for a patient in need. I also just learned that two more matches were made from the various bone marrow drives we held for William. Three potential lifesaving matches, that's pretty amazing!

November 24

We made it to Houston and beat the rain. We looked at one apartment and went ahead and got it. Now we have a temporary home in Houston and don't have to keep calling weekly and praying there is an available hotel within fifteen miles of MDA. I don't even know the address here yet. It wasn't supposed to be ready until Tuesday so I will sign a lease tomorrow and get all that. The ride down here wore William out and he has been asleep for several hours.

Hopefully when he wakes up he will feel like exploring the apartment. He was not at all looking forward to making this move because he feels like he has lost all his freedoms and is tied to the hospital. He is so miserable, feeling so dependent on others for everything. I hope that with having an actual apartment verses a hotel room, he feels more at home. Hopefully.

November 25

Okay Folks, here it is...his insurance denied the transplant again. They want a more detailed treatment plan along with William's medical history and physical. It completely and totally pisses me off! They have this information! The doctor said he will submit everything they are asking for again, but they are being vague as to exactly what they want and he feels they are stalling because they don't want to pay the $1.2 million procedure.

My first step is to reach out for some political help, and news media. Then I plan to post the insurance phone number and turn you guys loose afterward. We will be doing some fundraisers as well. I am also asking the hospital what our other options are if they keep denying. I don't know if this is normal or not, but if it's a fight they want...they got it!

> Comment 2: What a bunch of assholes. I can't stand it!! God bless you all dealing with this on top of everything. Why do they bother? They are going to end up having to pay for it and they KNOW it!! The best place to start is to contact the employer who's carrying the plan (unless it's an individual plan) and let them know about the denial, and have their broker push the claim through. I think

that he should apply for social security disability, and he will probably be denied, and then once he's denied, apply for Medicaid as a secondary insurance. Keep pushing the hospital to do the transplant, and they should proceed as planned. It will all come together, this is bull. I can't believe they are putting you through this. I'm so sorry.

Comment 5: So sorry! This pissed me off too! Probably everyone who reads this is, this doesn't make any sense at all and I'm continuing to pray and whatever I can do to help I Will! ((Hugs))

Comment 8: Contact your senator & the media. Give us their number. It appears that in order to get. what he needs, there must be a loudness that cannot be ignored. Make them explain to the public why they are denying this procedure! It's much easier for cowards such as these to deny a heartbroken family than an enraged public!

Comment 12: I would contact your congressman for help! Then take your problem to the media, & have them check into why the Dr & Insurance Co isn't doing anything!!! After all it's about HEALTH INSURANCE & YOUR CHILD!!! If it was me I would be all over them like flies on dodo!!!

Comment 14: Get an attorney that specialized in "bad faith" against insurance companies. It won't cost you to talk to one and some will work on a % basis of a settlement (hopefully it won't go that far). Insurance co's guilty of bad faith have to pay TREBLE damages. They hate the phrase "bad faith" and a letter from a lawyer just may do the trick. It's worth a try...

Comment 29: I'm happy to put a 1-800 number on speed dial to my left and my Keurig to my right. My husband says I will drive a point into the ground, just to see how far it will go....just turn me loose....

Comment 30: What Deborah said !!!!! ME TOO !!!!!!! You go Amy .... kick some ass !!!!

Comment 31: I'm sorry they denied again, but if you post the # I have all the time in the world to call..and I will repost to my friends and some of them have time to call all day too. whatever I can do to help

Comment 40: Escalate. Use whatever avenue you can find. Surely there are organizations that can help. Call the N.I.H., call the news people, your senator... and we'll keep praying. Love you.

Comment 68: Let me know when you come up with a plan. I'm in. We WILL beat this. Tell him I love him.

November 27

I have to say thank you to a friend of mine, Candice for composing this letter and explanation as to what is happening to William, and for posting it on her page as a "call to arms!" I am so exhausted I can't even compose my thoughts right now.

To be honest, she wrote this so beautifully, there is nothing I could say to make it better or clearer. So please read this post, share it, and take action. The addresses and e-mails or phone numbers to where you can call/write/email to help William are listed. Thank you all so much for your help. Together we are going to move this mountain!

"Day 108 After Aidan Went Home URGENT---PLEASE READ---I need every one of you to please read this, to help, to like, to share...Basically, I need help moving a mountain, and I've seen what the collective spirit of Aidan's One Love community is capable of in the past. I have been doing my best to avoid the holidays as these first ones without Aidan make his absence so obvious that every minute is a little longer than it seems like it should be and every minute hurts a little more than it seems like it should. For that reason, I'm doing my best to avoid and skip the holidays this year (not the spiritual part, just the store-bought-festive-being-merry-around-people part) and that has included stepping away from my blog for a little bit and giving my time to people and causes I can help. But today, I am back. Today, I need to tell you guys a story and then I need to issue a plea for action-a call to arms of sorts. There is a young man named William Purdom, and he just recently turned 21 on Halloween. I was introduced to his mom, Amy, in June of this year when William was diagnosed with T Cell ALL (Acute Lymphocytic Leukemia). I have both her pleas and permission to post this today. T-Cell ALL is rare, generally aggressive, and fairly tricky in its attack. It is usually resistant to chemotherapy. It very often requires a bone marrow (stem cell) transplant. And in William's case, just like with my precious Aidan, transplant is his ONLY hope for survival. It took months to get this kid into remission. Chemo after chemo failed. Does this sound familiar? That was Aidan. Finally, just recently, William reached remission. He is physically ready for his transplant. The window of opportunity is short. He must transplant before his leukemia learns how to resist the medicine; and given a small amount of time, it will. Just last month, more good news: there is a PERFECT MATCH from an anonymous donor out there waiting to donate the life-saving stem cells! And now to the terrible part of this message and where you can truly help save this kid's life: WILLIAM'S INSURANCE (managed health care plan) HAS DENIED HIS TRANSPLANT. TWICE. When he was age 20 and covered by traditional Medicaid, the transplant was approved to be paid in full as a medical necessity for survival. When he turned 21 a month ago, he was forced off traditional Medicaid which covers kids and moved onto a managed care Medicaid, at which point the transplant was re-evaluated by the new provider and denied. You guys, my job here is not to get into a political or moral discussion here about healthcare, Medicaid, managed care Medicaid, etc. My goal is to tell you very simple facts in a way that is hopefully easy to understand. William's transplant which was approved through traditional Medicaid has been denied through Managed Care Medicaid which he was forced to move to because he was 21. The reason for the denial is being listed as: "Experimental and Not Medically Necessary." There are two truths to the denial overall, but NEITHER is an actual reason for the denial. Truth 1) All stem cell transplants are "experimental." Transplant will only yield a 50% survival rate, so yeah, technically that is experimental. However, the mortality (death) rate is 100% without it. Truth 2) Not medically necessary. Of course transplant isn't medically necessary on a dead person. But it is INHERENTLY WRONG to call a transplant "Not Medically Necessary" due to the disease being a terminal illness when the transplant is the ONLY thing that can make the disease not only no longer terminal-but CURED. Yes, it's only a 50/50 chance. I know as well as only a person who's gone through the ups and downs of leukemia, chemo, and transplant that the cure sometimes also kills. Transplant is a hard road to walk down, and your kid might still go home to fly and love even after all the effort is made. But I fiercely believe that if it is William's turn to "make the trip up to heaven" as 80 would say, it should be because the Lord calls him. NOT BECAUSE THE INSURANCE COMPANY SAID NO. The only thing that changed here is William's age (and because of that, his Medicaid). I promise you, it doesn't matter if your baby is 6 years old, 21 years old, or 60 years old. To ride the leukemia roller coaster, to constantly hear "I'm sorry, he's failed to achieve remission and we can't transplant without it and he will die soon without transplant," and to hold on strong to your faith in the midst of it is HARD. But as chemo parents, as "Mom-Cologists," THAT'S WHAT WE DO. And many of us get very good at it. But to keep the faith, to get to that point which seemed so unlikely-remission...and your child's body is ready for transplant, and the insurance says "Denied" is unthinkable. William is being seen by the top T Cell ALL specialists in the United States. His care is based out of MD Anderson. He's not sitting in some hokey hospital being diagnosed by a first year resident. He has FIVE recommendations from the top specialists in the country telling the provider that death is the definite outcome for this patient without the procedure. -------------- I didn't wake up one day and say, "hey, I think I'm going to become an activist. I think I'm going to lobby and advocate for patient's rights." I did wake up today, as I will every day for the rest of my life, without my son. And it hurts and it sucks and I would trade anything for five more minutes with him. But I am blessed with the peace of knowing WE DID EVERY SINGLE BIG AND LITTLE THING WE COULD TO SAVE HIM. It was his time to go home, and that was abundantly clear when I was out of earthly options to keep him here with me. William is NOT out of options. His Mom shouldn't have to wake up one single day wondering if her baby would be here if only he would have gotten his transplant. That is a pain I cannot imagine, and that is a reality I cannot allow without giving my above-ground effort to change the decision. I know that I alone am easy to ignore. But many of us together can make that "no" a "yes." We can move a mountain. I've seen it happen before. I'm going to list several agencies and emails plus regular addresses. Please write to them and either use the accurate info I've listed here about William and his case or just copy and paste the following letter:

Subject Line: William Purdom Transplant Denial

To Whom it May Concern: This letter is to express my utmost concern for a violation of patient rights by Managed Care Medicaid in the case of 21 year old William Purdom. William is being treated for T-Cell ALL and his only hope for survival is a bone marrow/stem cell transplant. He was originally approved for the procedure as a medical necessity under traditional Medicaid, but has now been denied after becoming an adult and being forced to move to the managed care Medicaid with the reasoning of "not a medical necessity/experimental." William is being seen by the top T Cell ALL specialists in the United States. His care is based out of MD Anderson. He's not sitting in a county hospital being diagnosed by a first year resident. He has FIVE recommendations from the top specialists in the country telling the provider that death is the definite outcome for this patient without the procedure. I ask that you review this case and PLEASE ACT NOW to right this grave injustice towards this young patient and his family. Each day that William does not receive the life-saving transplant, he is that much closer to losing his life. William deserves the chance of life that this transplant can give him. PLEASE ACT NOW. Kind regards, ----------------------

Here is a list of places you can send your letter (and I've been advised that email is best-and if you accidentally send it multiple times...oops. But it will be seen): Complaints for Managed Health Plan HPM_complaints@hhsc.state.tx.us Texas Dept of Insurance Consumer protection mail code 111-1A Consumerprotection@tdi.state.tx.us PO Box 149104 Austin, TX 78714 Senator Ted Cruz 300 E 8th, suite 961 Austin, TX 78710 512-916-5834 Website to find out local representatives and their contact information www.fyi.legis.state.tx.us ---------------------------

On this day before Thanksgiving, I'm so grateful for every one of you and the love and support you CONSTANTLY show my child and me. When I needed financial help for Lucie, you were there with pure love and generosity. Today I need you to help me campaign for this family. If there's ANY chance, especially a 50/50 chance that they can celebrate their next Thanksgiving with every member of their family sitting around the table, don't they deserve it? Thank you so very much. Thank you for LIKING and SHARING this post. And for asking your friends to Like and Share. Thank you for your ACTIONS of sending messages to those who have the ability to turn this "no" into a resounding "YES." We can do it. ----------------------
Today's picture is June 13, 2013-the day of Aidan's bone marrow transplant. It was a happy day full of hope and faith and gratitude. William and his family deserve this day too. Love and blessings, Candice Lawson"

> *Comment 1: I will be spending some time this weekend now that I know who to contact!! This is so well written and perfectly to the point!*
>
> *Comment 4: Just sent the letter to all 31 State*

Senators, David Dewhurst, and Rick Perry and to the emails listed above....and will do so till they act!!!!

Comment 5: Will get this out as much as I can as I also shared it on my facebook and will tweet the info out as soon as I can figure out how to link to the post....You're in my prayers

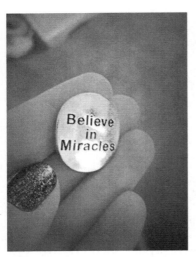

November 28

I feel as though I am walking through a very dark valley. Last night I cried myself to sleep, praying for a miracle. And to be honest I don't care how it comes! Transplant, miracle drug or a touch from God and a miracle healing, I don't care! I just want my son back and want this horrible cancer out of him!

Dr. Alvarado told me Monday that William is in a very critical place. They MUST do everything possible to keep him in remission. If his cancer comes back, they will abandon the current regimen and go to the next option, but there will much less chance he will go back into remission. We are racing the clock with a super aggressive cancer. Dr. Alvarado said if this happens, we will be in "much deeper and much darker waters."

His stem cell doctor told me yesterday they need to strengthen William but keep him in remission at the same time. He is on ridiculous amounts of chemo to keep his cancer away, but at the same time the chemo is breaking William down. His liver is showing more signs of damage so he had to be removed from two of his medications. It's a very fine balancing act. Dr. Champlin said they will work on the appeal and get it submitted (again) and he asked me to keep rallying the troops for public appeal! It will work! If you missed yesterday's post here are the places you can write, call or email on William's behalf:

Complaints for Managed Health Plan
HPM_complaints@hhsc.state.tx.us
Texas Dept of Insurance
Consumer protection mail code 111-1A
PO Box 149104 Austin, TX 78714
Consumerprotection@tdi.state.tx.us

Senator Ted Cruz
300 E 8th, suite 961
Austin, TX 78710
512-916-5834

Rep. Jeb Hensarling
2228 Rayburn HOB
Washington, D.C. 20515
Phone: (202) 225-3484

Website to find out local representatives and their contact information www.fyi.legis.state.tx.us

In yesterday's post, Candice even went as far as to create a sample letter, if you so choose to, use it. It has all the pertinent information included and is well written.

Trust me, I was so angry that when I filed my complaint I told them "it appeared to me that whoever is making this decision has their head shoved up their ass and it's about time they remove it!" I also asked the name of the person who keeps denying him, because *when* my son dies, I am going to have their name listed on his death certificate as the "Cause of Death!"

I think Candice's words are much more appropriate; HOWEVER I did get a response! Two actually, with very detailed information that they want to see so I was able to give that information to Dr. Champlin. If you want to use Candice's letter here it is:

Subject Line: William Purdom Transplant Denial

To Whom it May Concern:

This letter is to express my utmost concern for a violation of patient rights by Managed Care Medicaid, in the case of 21 year old William Purdom. William is being treated for T-Cell ALL and his only hope for survival is a bone marrow/stem cell transplant. He was originally approved for the procedure as a medical necessity under traditional Medicaid, but has now been denied after becoming an adult and being forced to move to a managed care Medicaid, with the reasoning of "not a medical necessity/experimental." William is being seen by the top T Cell ALL specialists in the United States. His care is based out of MD Anderson. He's not sitting in a county hospital being diagnosed by a first year resident. He has FIVE recommendations from the top specialists in the country telling the provider that death is the definite outcome for this patient without the procedure. I ask that you review this case and PLEASE ACT NOW to right this grave injustice towards this young patient and his family.

Each day that William does not receive the life-saving transplant, he is that much closer to losing his life. William deserves the chance of life that this transplant can give him. PLEASE ACT NOW.

Kind regards,

Candice also sent me this picture this morning. She found it yesterday while cleaning and didn't know where it came from. She reminded me to believe in miracles, and keep my faith even in the hard times. I needed these words because my tank is empty right now. I am weary and tired, but I look at my warrior son, and I will keep going. He is fighting a good fight, and I will stand with him and fight with him...all the way to our miracle!

November 30

William had a very good day. He has been up and out of his wheelchair, walking around strong and stable. He even cooked his own breakfast! I love the good days. We are praying and holding on for a miracle. I hope this coming week brings the news we need the most. Keep writing, calling and emailing. I have contacted Fox 4 and depending on the outcome of the next appeal, we will start media coverage if needed.

December 1

I am back at home. I decorated for Christmas today, and it's a little bitter-sweet. I am not in the Christmas spirit right now, but I am also trying to maintain some sense of normalcy for James and Abbey. My parents are in

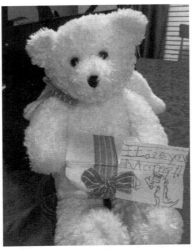

Houston with William this week while I take care of Abbey. She is having dental surgery in a few days.

While unpacking boxes I ran across this angel bear. William gave it to me one Christmas when he was very young, about five or six, judging by the note enclosed. He used to get my Post-it notes and leave me notes all over the house or my office. I still have several of them. While I hope he gets the approval soon, and the transplant as quickly as possible, it's hard to imagine not having him at home for Christmas this year! It's even harder knowing that if he doesn't get this transplant, this will be my last Christmas with him ever.

December 2

You know those days when everything goes wrong? William is having that day today. They got to the hospital at 9:00 a.m. for lab checks and chemo, and it is now 5:45 p.m. and he has another seven-plus hours to go! He also needs blood, which makes me nervous after the last blood transfusion reaction. But he is in the best possible place and I know that, but still 16 hours at the hospital is hard, even on a healthy person.

December 3

William ended up being at the hospital for 18 1/2 hours yesterday! He is not doing well today at all, simply from pure exhaustion. He received two units of blood and chemo yesterday. I would greatly appreciate extra prayers for comfort and rest for him.

He goes back on Thursday for another blood check and possible transfusions if his numbers continue to drop. Please remember that cancer patients (especially leukemia patients) require considerable amounts of blood and platelets to stay alive. Give blood, and give often!

December 4

I wanted to pass along an update on the insurance denial situation. First, let me say thank you for all the calls, emails and letters on William's behalf. Both from this page and my friend, Candice's page (One Love for 80). The support for William has been amazing! My phone has rung non-stop for three days now. I am hearing that things are moving "in the right direction." I also talked with MDA today and they should be resubmitting the appeal today or first thing in the morning. Dr. Champlin was in a meeting and they wanted him to give it the final "once over" to make sure it was perfect before submission.

I am working closely with the Texas Department of Insurance, Sen. Bob Deuell's office and several other entities as well as a few "angels" in Austin who are helping too. Once again, we just need to pray for his insurance company to approve the transplant. I expect to hear something next week, so I will keep you updated once I do.

Right now, William is hanging in there. He got Vincristine (one of the harder chemos) on Monday and he gets it again on the 9th. Mom and Dad are with him in Houston and it looks like the weather will keep them there until late next week. His spirits are good, and he is staying strong.

Thanks everyone! I am hoping some very good news is just around the corner!

December 5

We have received the miracle we have been praying for! I got the call from the insurance company that they have approved William's transplant! About thirty minutes after they called, a representative from Senator Bob Deuell's office called to be sure I heard the news. He told me that Sen. Deuell demanded that the insurance company call me personally to let me know they had approved William. Thank you all so much for your calls, emails and letters. They made a difference! Thank you for your support, prayers and encouragement as well. These have been very difficult weeks but you have all helped us get through. Now we wait for some paperwork to be finalized and then will hear when to expect the transplant procedure to begin.

WE DID IT! WE MOVED A MOUNTAIN! It took the strength and faith of us all, but together we did it!

> Comment 5: Thank God!!!! So happy that you finally got the approval and can save your worries for taking care of William and not stupid bureaucratic insurance ridiculousness!! They knew they had to approve it from the start, I hate that they put you all through all that. Time to get those healthy cells!! YAY!!

> Comment 19: Praise God from whom all blessings flow! Continued prayers!

Comment 26: AWESOMENESS!!!!!

Comment 34: Now that's an awesome Christmas present!

Comment 41: So exited, elated, jubilant, ecstatic, thrilled, joyful, etc. for all of you! Now everyone can spend their energy getting William through this transplant! stay warm, stay safe, stay healthy...

Comment 43: AWESOMENESS!!!!! This just took my crazy, stress-filled day and turned it into a JOYOUS ONE....I am CELEBRATING with you!!!!!!!!!!!!!!!!!

December 6

A couple of Christmas Angels came to visit William yesterday. While he was spending his day at the hospital with Mom and Dad, our dear friend Denise and her daughter, Laura went into the apartment and decorated for Christmas. William was very surprised when he got back.

Today we found out William will hopefully be getting a break from the chemo so he can rest and gain strength in preparation for his transplant. He has to get more Vincristine on Monday, but the hope is, that will be his last round of out-patient chemo until he is ready to be admitted for the transplant. This means several things; he will get stronger and feel better, have to take fewer medications and allow his body to rest and that we can all be together on Christmas. We will have a better idea of his upcoming schedule after the donor is contacted. We should know more by next week, but for now I am one incredibly happy Mama!

December 7

It's funny how God works in your life and you don't realize it until later. I have mentioned Denise before (it was her and her daughter that brought the Christmas tree for William) but let me tell you how we met. Last year, just after Christmas, Denise and her daughter Laura found a young male beagle that had been thrown from a car and was injured. They took him to the shelter and ended up fostering him when his owners wouldn't come back for him. Just a couple months later in February of this year, my husband and I decided it was time to get a playmate for Lucy, our very energetic and mischievous beagle. Her doggy friend had died and Lucy was left alone. Through a Facebook connection we were introduced to Denise, and ended up adopting Linus. We were happy to have Linus and even happier to have found a new friend as well.

Just a little over three months after meeting Denise, William was diagnosed. Denise immediately called me and said I needed to get him to MD Anderson. She opened her home to us, has taken us to MDA and met with the doctors with us, taken notes to make sure we have the information right, donated platelets for William, and brought us apple pie when he is inpatient, and so much more!

The way I see it, God knew we would need and Angel in Houston to help us get through this, so He used a dog to bring two families together. Denise is not just a friend; she is much, much more! Denise is forever part of our family. We love you Denise!

December 8

Y'all please say a prayer for William. Mom and Dad are taking him to the ER now. He has a fever, extreme weakness and pains that are different from the "normal" pains he has been having. I will update once I know more.

Update: I just spoke with the ER nurse. William's white blood cell counts are hovering just above zero so he has no immune system right now. He has a fast heart rate, fever, vomiting and he is coughing. He has "something" but they are not sure exactly what. They are looking specifically for RSV (a virus). It will take 24 hours to get the blood cultures back to know exactly what he has, but they have started him on broad spectrum antibiotics for now. More than likely he will be admitted to the hospital since he is neutropenic and symptomatic. When the doctor comes in we will know more. He isn't thrilled but he is using the internet to do some Christmas shopping for his little brother and sister to pass the time. And he said there won't be any noisy neighbors to wake him up (our apartment neighbors are horrible and wake him up every night).

December 9

William quit throwing up and was able to hold some food down today. The pain seems to be subsiding as well, according to my dad. He did get a blood transfusion this morning. His hemoglobin took a substantial drop in just a few hours. They will keep an eye on the blood counts and continue to transfuse as he needs. His white count is still hovering just above zero, so no improvement there. They are waiting on the results from the blood cultures but don't believe they will reveal much. The antibiotics they have him on will kill any kind of infection whether bacterial, viral or fungal.

He was supposed to get chemo today but due to his low counts, mystery infection and other symptoms his doctor felt it would be best to wait till Thursday. It's a particularly nasty chemo and he needs time to recover before they "hit" him and knock him down again. At this point, no one has mentioned how long he will have to stay inpatient. He hates being there too. Just hates it!

We are hoping to have a date soon for his transplant. It depends on the donor schedule at this point. I will be glad when he gets the break from chemo. It is so hard on the body! I teased him last night and asked him, "Why did you have to go and get so sick?" He replied, "Well THEY'RE the ones that keep pumping me full of poison!" Even when sick, he holds on to that sense of humor!

December 10

William is very weak today. His hemoglobin has dropped again, even after the blood transfusion yesterday so he will get more blood today. Dr. Alvarado just left and he said what is happening, is that William has endured such toxic levels of chemo for such an extended period of time that his body is just no longer strong enough to fight off the effects. He is still due for another dose of chemo this week but Dr. Alvarado wants to closely monitor his blood counts and symptoms and hold off administering this chemo until it becomes absolutely necessary. William is just too weak to take it, and the effects could be devastating to him. He will continue to stay in the hospital for now.

His stem cell doctor would prefer he gets no more chemo at all so he can be strong when he goes in for the transplant, but his leukemia doctor has to closely monitor him to make sure his cancer doesn't return. It is a very fine balancing act, and they are working closely together. If he can stop the chemo now without his cancer returning, then he might be able to be home for Christmas to see all his family and friends before going in for his transplant. I know that would lift his spirits tremendously.

While you are praying for William, I would also ask that you pray for a friend of William's, Gary. Gary is also at MDA and is inpatient as well. He is preparing for his stem cell transplant right now, and will get it Friday. Gary is an amazing man, and he has been a great friend and support for William. They met shortly after William was diagnosed and have walked most of this journey together. It's pretty cool that they both are getting their transplants about the same time, so they will be going through recovery together too, and can help support each other through the next step in this journey.

December 11

William is still in a lot of pain but Dr. Alvarado feels it is from the chemo and low blood counts. They have put his chemo on hold for now so he can recover. As his counts improve and the chemo wears off, the pain will dissipate. They are hoping the transplant will be soon enough that he will not have to take any more chemo until he is admitted for the transplant. We are waiting to hear from the transplant team regarding a date, but for now William just needs time to rest, recover and build strength.

December 12

Yes! Little glimmers of hope! William's white cells have cratered, but his hemoglobin and platelets have started on an upward trend. He is still neutropenic and is susceptible to any and all infections, but his body is beginning to recover. Yay! His pain is getting more manageable and if he continues to improve over the next 24 hours he will be released from the hospital tomorrow. If he is able to reasonably manage his pain, his doctor has even given the ok for him to come home (back to Dallas) for the weekend. Keep those healing prayers coming.

December 13

Well, no such luck! William's hemoglobin dropped again and he ended up getting another blood transfusion today, so no discharge. He might get to leave the hospital tomorrow. The doctor wanted to wait another day and see how he does. He is not feeling good so more than likely he will not feel like traveling home, even if they let him go.

December 14

William finally broke out of the hospital! His blood counts stayed up overnight so the doctor let him go. He didn't feel strong enough to make the four hour drive back home so we are staying at the apartment. If he continues to improve and get stronger, he should be able to be home for Christmas. We see the stem cell doctor, Dr. Champlin, this Thursday and should have an update on the transplant date.

December 15

Today the sun was shining bright and William and I were able to get out of the apartment for a little bit and enjoy it. He is doing much better, walking steady and strong. He didn't need his wheel chair or cane today at all. After we ran a few errands we came back to the apartment and have been watching Christmas movies all day . He really wants to be home for Christmas, and then he is ready to get this transplant underway. Now that we know William has no infections, and he is stronger, we are going to visit Gary tomorrow. He is on day +2 from his transplant.

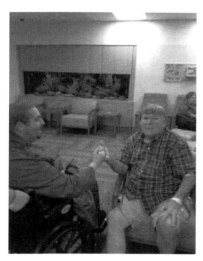

December 16

William, my family, and I are heartbroken this morning. We are devastated to learn that our dear friend, Gary, lost his fight this morning at 5:08 a.m. He apparently developed a strep infection, and it went to his heart. I just can't believe he is gone!

William is taking the news hardest of all. To lose a friend is hard enough, but to lose a cancer friend is even worse. There is a bond between cancer friends that runs much deeper than most. Gary and William were supposed to fight this beast together, help each other recover and celebrate their new lives with a big ole' Texas style BBQ party once they were both able to return home.

Gary will be greatly missed. He was a prayer warrior and a devoted friend. Our loss is Heaven's gain! Gary loved The Lord our God with all his heart, and he is resting now in His everlasting arms.

Welcome to My Kingdom

You knew right away when it was your last day
Your pain eased
You suffered no more
And you caught a glimpse of angels galore

You settled upon a pair of wings
Feeling those white, feathery, beautiful things
You flew with the angels and after the flight
You stopped at the golden gates shining so bright

Here, the Lord welcomed you with His warm embrace
You even felt warmth in the smile on His face
He said, "Welcome to My Kingdom my dear son
Your heavy heart must weigh a ton"
From all the suffering you went through
You knew what He said was true

So He took you by the hand
And led you through the Heavenly land
You listened to the birds and gazed at the flowers and trees
And felt a sense of joy and peace

You looked down from up above
And reassured the ones you love
"I am with God walking around
But better yet, I am in His presence forever safe and
sound"

by Benny DiFranco

Comment 4: So sorry for your incredible loss. I'm so glad your paths led you both together for encouragement and strength. I know he left an indelible mark on your life and I know you find comfort in knowing you will see him again someday. Prayers going up for you and his family during this difficult time.

Comment 35: Gary is your cheerleader in heaven now. He will personally take you to the throne room daily. We love you so much.

December 17

William had some lab work today, and it was sad to be at MDA and know that Gary isn't here, and that he won't be any more. It seems a little lonelier now, not just the hallways and waiting rooms at MDA, but the whole journey. Gary's funeral is on Friday back home, and if all goes well we should be able to make it. Actually, there is no "should" about it, William told me IS going, no matter what! With or without the doctor's permission to travel!

We have to watch and be careful right now. Some of William's counts have bounced back nicely but his white cells are barely budging. He is still neutropenic and had some mild chest pains today with a rapid heartbeat. They are watching closely for pneumonia since he is prone to getting it. On Thursday he will have another blood check to monitor his counts and have a CT scan of his lungs. Hopefully we will have an update on the transplant too.

December 18

If all goes well tomorrow, William and I will be heading back home for Christmas. He has a cough and had some very minor chest pain on Tuesday, so we are doing a CT scan of his lungs in the morning just to be sure he doesn't have pneumonia again. He is prone to it and usually has no symptoms when it comes on. His heart rate has been high for several days, so we need to keep a close eye on that too when we are back home. But he has been out of his wheelchair for two solid days now, walking without a cane or anything for support or balance, so that's good news.

He told me today he is nervous and worried his cancer will come back before the transplant. He said at first he could handle the chemo but there was a turning point where he said he could feel a difference. He could feel it killing him. He is worried if his cancer returns he will have to do more chemo and may not be strong enough going into his transplant. I am scared of the same thing too, to be honest. Turns out we have both been counting the weeks since he has been off chemo and keeping an eye on it. Evidently his leukemia doctor is as well. Dr. Alvarado is on vacation but he called me tonight to tell me he has limited access to email but he is keeping up with William, and he just wanted to touch base with me to check on him. He really doesn't want him to have any more chemo if at all possible. He told William that he was surprised he lasted this long considering the doses they have had him on! But it was necessary because of how aggressive his cancer was.

I am very thankful for good doctors, and caring doctors! I know William is in good hands, even though I am scared too. I also know William is in God's hands. I can almost hear Gary saying, "It ain't nothin' but a thang. We got Jesus so it'll be alright!"

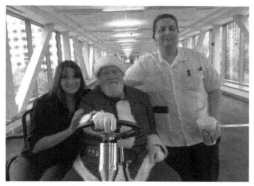

December 19

We are heading HOME for Christmas!

December 20

I have much to talk about today. We are home now. I sent yesterday's message while sitting at a red light so I couldn't give you all the information I wanted to.

WE HAVE A TRANSPLANT DATE! William's physical birthday will always be October 31, but his re-birthday will be January 15 if all goes well. This date could change; there are a lot of factors that play into it. He will be going several weeks without chemo, and if his cancer decides to return it will push his date back, so we need to immerse him in prayers of protection starting now. Also, a small infection could push his date back as well. Again, prayers of protection.

We have limited information on his donor. She is 35 years old, very healthy, a committed donor. She possibly may live overseas (they couldn't tell us specifically to help protect her privacy), and her blood type is A+ so William's blood type will change. Our coordinator will ask her if she has any food allergies or other allergies that we need to be aware of, to help make this grafting process easier, as

William will lose all of his current allergies and adopt hers. She will be donating her actual bone marrow to him, not the stem cells. This will lessen the risk of Graft vs. Host Disease (GVHD) but it will take a little bit longer to graft, so it may require an extra week in the hospital. It's a good trade off though. GVHD sucks and is no fun! We do not have her name, but I ask you to pray earnestly for her as well. God knows who she is, even if we do not!

I also have a very important request of you, MD Anderson is critically low on blood, and they have to ration transfusions right now! They use more blood than any hospital in the nation, over 600 units of blood products daily. Cancer patients depend on blood and platelets to survive. Leukemia patients make up over 80% of the total blood transfusions they give. Donated blood and platelets have kept William alive for six months. I am so grateful to all the people who donate. But the holiday season is full of shopping, parties and traveling. We get busy and don't make time to donate blood. Cancer doesn't take Christmas off! The need is every day; I want to ask you to please make some time to donate blood before Christmas. If you live in or near Houston, you can go to MD Anderson.

Part of the ration process means people will not get the blood they need, even the children. Whole blood and platelets are needed. If you have two hours, please consider platelets. It is better for a patient to receive a unit of platelets that was pulled from a single source. Normally they pull platelets out of several whole blood donations and have to make a "mixed bag" effect, but this increases the patient's chance of reactions.

Employers, please consider offering an incentive for your team to donate. Perhaps offer an extra hour for lunch or a recognition program...just something! Hold a drive at your place of business. Every drop of blood that is donated will save a life. Now if that doesn't build team spirit and lift morale then what does?

If you are not able to give at MDA, then find your local hospital or blood bank, but please just donate. I do it myself. I am not a fan of needles either, but I do it and so can you. Be a hero today! If you are in Houston, I am donating again on December 27, meet me there and we'll do it together!

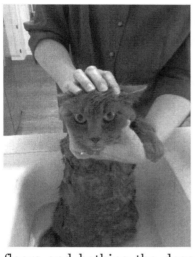

December 22

The last couple days have been busy. Part of being neutropenic means EVERYTHING in the house has to be cleaned! This includes the animals. Yesterday and today have been spent cleaning and sterilizing, wiping all door handles, faucets, knobs and light switches with bleach water, steam cleaning the floors and bathing the dogs and the cat. While the cat looks mad, she actually handles bath time pretty well. Once when William was in the second grade, Noel jumped in the bathtub with him. She is a very unique cat!

We attended Gary's funeral on Friday, and it was an amazing celebration of his life, and his love for people and for his Savior. We had met some of his family already, but had the privilege to meet the rest of the family. Once again, our family has grown even bigger. Cancer can be very ugly and it can be a constant reminder of pain and sorrow, but it has a brighter side too. Because of this journey, we have met some of the most amazing people and formed friendships that are stronger than most, and will stay with us for the rest of our lives. Even in the midst of the trial, we are still being blessed!

December 23

Wow! I just saw William's updated schedule for December 27 through January 8, when he is admitted to prep for the transplant. He is going to have just about every possible test run on him. He will have CT scans of his sinuses and lungs, several different heart tests, lumbar punctures, anesthesia tolerance, and blood tests - you name it! He has some very long days ahead full of poking, prodding, sticking, drilling and scanning!

We also will be moving to a different apartment. I mentioned the noise from the upstairs neighbors, but it just got to the point we weren't able to sleep at night and it didn't matter how many times we called security and the apartment manager, there was no improvement. So a friend helped us and found a possible new place. If it works out it will be a little closer to the hospital and be a substantial savings over the current place. Now it really feels like things are falling into place.

I think we are ready for Christmas. The house is clean and sterilized, the animals are all bathed, the gifts have been sprayed with Lysol and wrapped (not joking), and I have a head start on the cooking. It's amazing the precautions we have to take right now to keep William from catching anything. I went to pick up a prescription for him today at Tom Thumb and when I walked in the door I heard several people coughing so I immediately put my mask on. Normally hearing someone cough wouldn't even faze me, but I am much more aware of things like that now, especially being in a group or large crowd. My favorite part is how people cut a wide a girth to avoid me as if I am the contagious one when I wear a mask! Ha-ha little do they know its *them* I am trying to avoid! But whatever works, that's all that matters.

Tomorrow is Christmas Eve, and I hope everyone enjoys your time with family and friends. When it comes down to it, the time you get to spend with those you love is the best gift, and what lasting memories are made of! And may God comfort those who are missing loved ones this Christmas season.

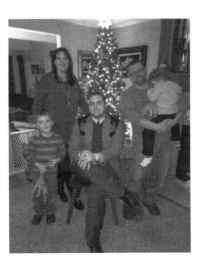

December 25

Wishing you all a Merry Christmas! Thank you for your prayers, love, support and encouragement over these last six months. You have helped me get through some very rough times, and held me together when I felt like falling apart. This year I realize more than ever before just how blessed I am, blessed that my son is still with us to celebrate Christmas and blessed to have so many faithful friends and loved ones!

December 27

We are back at MDA for a battery of tests today. The lumbar puncture didn't go so well, so his doctor put him back in the wheelchair for the day. He doesn't want him up walking around. William has a herniated disk, and now has scar tissue that has developed, which tends to make the lumbar punctures more challenging and painful. He has also started getting hiccups every time he gets a lumbar puncture. Deep, painful hiccups that lasts for hours upon hours. We found an unusual cure for them. Another cancer mom suggested that he put a teaspoon of table sugar on his tongue, as far back as he can get it. Then drink a glass of water quickly. I don't know why this works, but it does!

Right now he is having three different tests on his heart and then off for a couple more appointments to finish off the day.

We looked at a couple of apartments yesterday. The one I was hoping would be perfect isn't going to work out. It was on the second floor and too far from the elevator. That mom-radar inside me was not at peace with it. I just kept thinking if there was a fire, there is no way he could get out in time, especially if he were in his wheelchair. So we looked at another place with an available ground-level apartment, and found one that works for us. It is smaller than our last apartment but it's quiet. No noisy neighbors!

We are moving right along towards transplant now. We just need to pray for his cancer not to return, for him not to get sick or be exposed to any infections, for the process to run smoothly and of course for his donor. Right now his life is directly connected to hers.

December 28

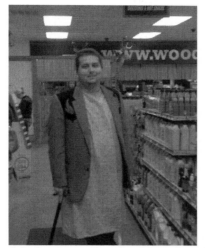

We came back home last night since this was William's last chance to come home for several months. So here is William adorned in his fashionable hospital gown and a sports coat. The trip was hard on him after the lumbar puncture and fashion was the least of his concerns. If you know him, you know this is a new low for him since he is always dressed up.

The trip ended up being too much for him and William is in a lot of pain right now. He has asked me to post for him and request for no visitors. He is hurting and needs to rest for his return trip and the procedures that lay ahead. Please limit phone calls today as well; maybe tomorrow he will feel like taking calls again. Thank you for understanding and keeping William's health and care a top priority.

December 30

I have an urgent prayer need for William. I received a call from his Stem Cell Team this morning, and the fluid from his spinal tap done on Friday has some inconclusive cells. They cannot tell if they are malignant so they need to re-do the spinal tap. Due to his herniated disk and scar tissue buildup (from the previous lumbar punctures), this is a very painful procedure for William. And of course, the obvious concern is that if the cells are malignant then it means his cancer has returned and is trying to attack his brain, as it tried before.

This just sucks! They will repeat the spinal tap tomorrow and we need to pray for the most skilled hands on the planet to do the procedure so there is no digging and rolling the needle around in his spine. We need to pray for his comfort during and after the procedure and pray the cells are *not* cancerous. He will also have a bone marrow aspiration this week so pray his bone marrow is also clear of cancer.

We knew going this long without chemo was a risk with the very aggressive nature of his cancer, but his body needed to rest and be strengthened before the transplant. Just please pray!

December 31

The spinal tap is done. We are back at the apartment and William is resting now. I am hoping for a very good report. The same gal did the spinal tap today as well as last Friday. She went into his spine in a different area trying to avoid the scar tissue and herniated disc. She said it looked cleaner and had no blood in it. This is a very good sign so hopefully we will get great news on Thursday, and his spinal fluid will be cancer free. If all goes well, his transplant will stay on schedule. No appointments tomorrow, so it will be a day to rest.

Thank you all for the prayers. They were definitely felt today. Happy and safe New Years, everyone. 2014 is going to be a great year! No more leukemia, no more cancer – just healing and restoration!

January 2

Who wants to hear some good news? The spinal fluid is negative for cancer/leukemia cells! Praise God! William had the bone marrow biopsy today, and his doctor will expedite those results, so we should have them Monday. Keep praying for no cancer!

Tomorrow will be another rough day. William goes in to have a subclavian catheter inserted and his PICC line removed. The catheter will run under his collar bone in his vein and into his heart valve. I am a little nervous about this. He will be completely put under for the procedure, he is very nervous about it too. There is a chance his lung could be punctured or collapsed so please keep those prayers coming. We had to watch a video explaining the insertion process and I just sat there fighting the need to vomit! Not that anything is wrong with the procedure itself, just that it's happening to my son. It still doesn't seem real sometimes.

We have to keep William isolated from the world right now. The transplant coordinator told us today that there are hundreds of cases of RSV and flu-strand-A in the hospital right now, so we all need to wear masks everywhere we go. To be safe, we need to keep William out of public places. William said we are living like hermits. Hey...whatever works!

January 3

William is done with the central line insertion and PICC line removal. He was ready to get out of there today. He has had a rough week with spinal taps, bone marrow biopsy and inserting this chest port. In his words, "My back hurts, my ass hurts, and my chest hurts! I just want to go home!"

Thankfully he has two days to rest with no appointments, and Monday will be a light day. He will be signing consent forms and meeting with his leukemia and stem cell doctors. Tuesday will be another long day, as they give him a small dose of chemo and measure how his body metabolizes it for the next 12 hours. This will help determine the maximum amount his body can tolerate for the conditioning process to get him ready for the bone marrow transplant. The chemo can cause seizures so I picked up some anti-seizure medicine for him to start taking on Monday.

For now I am just happy for the rest, even though I honestly feel restless and nervous. But at least maybe he will rest; he really needs it.

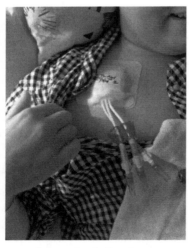

January 4

William is still a little sore from his chest catheter being inserted. As you can see it has three lumens hanging out of his chest. He said he feels like a cyborg. Since twenty-four hours have passed with no issues, we are out of the "danger zone" for punctured lungs or other complications, so that is a huge relief.

We haven't left the apartment today. We are doing everything we can to keep him isolated from people and possible infections. He is watching old reruns of *Scrubs* on

Netflix and I am watching a *Star Wars* marathon. I am glad for the time to rest for him. He has some very hard days ahead, starting Tuesday.

January 5

Today is my dad's birthday. Happy Birthday Daddy!

We will be back to the hospital tomorrow for William's last light day of appointments. The hard stuff begins on Tuesday with twelve hours of chemo and checking his blood, sometimes every fifteen minutes. This will help them determine the maximum amount of chemo his body can tolerate. Tuesday will be very hard on him! Then Wednesday he will be admitted to begin the conditioning process.

Part of me is excited and relieved, but there is also a scared part of me. I would be lying to you if I said there wasn't, especially after losing Gary only three days after his transplant. William's stem cell doctor reminded us last week that not everyone makes it. He said about 25% die. They are so matter-of-fact, the way they talk about death. Even though this has been my reality since June 6, 2013, it never gets easier to think about it. I know that without this transplant William has a 0% chance of survival. There was no way he could live with the aggressive nature of his cancer, so this transplant is giving him a second chance with a 75% success rate. It's not 100% and I wish it were, but I guess this is where faith steps in. My hope is not in percentages or doctors. Faith is the substance of things hoped for, the evidence of things not seen (Hebrews 11:1 NKJV).

January 6
Day -9 transplant

Did you notice the countdown? We have the green light to continue. The bone marrow biopsy came back with 3% leukemia blasts. This is up from the last test, but is okay to continue. Part of the conditioning process is high dose chemo which will kill any residual leukemia in William (as long as the blasts aren't too high).

We met with Dr. Alvarado, William's leukemia doctor, as kind of a farewell visit. It was almost sad to be honest. We have spent so much time with him over these past months, that it seems strange to be saying good bye. But I also found myself groping for answers again. I felt like I did seven months ago, wanting to know *WHY*, and if we have any idea *what* causes leukemia. The answers haven't changed. They still do not know what causes leukemia, though they think it may be linked to a virus but more research is needed.

We talked about the possibilities of William's leukemia being chronic versus acute, but in the end nothing would change. His cancer is so aggressive that the transplant is his only option. I think the scariest part of acute leukemia is that is can just happen to anyone, at any time with no warning! Finding the cause is the first step to finding the cure. Dr. Alvarado said much research is being done to discover that missing piece of the puzzle.

Tomorrow Dad will stay with William, and Mom and I are going to trade places. She has my younger two, and my five-year-old woke up crying for Mommy today, so I need to go back home and be with the little ones and my husband for a week and then return to Houston in time to be with William for the transplant. It is hard not to be able to be with all my kids at the same time. I wish I could be in two places at once! Mom and Dad will take good care of William; I just wish I could be here too. So please keep us all in your prayers tomorrow. Mom and I will be traveling, and William will be getting chemo and countless blood checks over a period of twelve hours. Please pray specifically that his veins stay nice and plump and don't collapse! This is very important to help him get through this test.

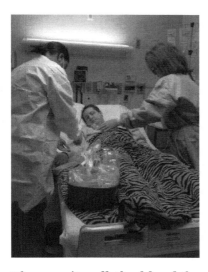

January 7
Day -8

It begins. They have started the Busulfan tolerance test. William just took Dilantin to help prevent seizures and at 9:30 a.m. will start the chemo dose. They will then pull blood for the next twelve hours, as often as every fifteen minutes. A very long day ahead!

They can't pull the blood from his port so he will have an IV stuck in his vein at the bend of his arm for over twelve hours, and he has to keep his arm straight during the entire time. If his veins collapse, they have to take it out and reinsert it into another vein.

January 8
Day -7

Today has been "hurry up and wait." Mom and Dad are still waiting on the call to bring him to the hospital to admit him. The admission office said it will probably be after 7:00 p.m. Tomorrow will begin the conditioning process for the actual transplant on January 15. The chemo is very strong and harsh. William's hair will fall out again, and he isn't happy about that. He told me when this is all over; he is growing his hair out again. He told me to prepare myself because he is planning on a Willie Nelson look. I say, why not? He earned it!

I can't believe we are one week away. In one week, he will get new his new bone marrow and his blood will begin to change over from A- to A+ (his donor's type). As her bone marrow and stem cells graph to his body, NEW blood will be made. Cancer free, leukemia free, NEW blood will flow through his veins!

During the last seven months, William and I have had many conversations. Some I have shared with you. But some of the things we have talked about I have kept private, partly because it may be deeply personal, and partly because some of the information is just too painful for me to write out, such as his "last wishes" if the worst were to happen. But there is a very special verse that we talked about one night on a drive back home from Houston. The verse is a promise, and a very personal promise for William.

"For I am about to do something new. See, I have already begun! Do you not see it? I will make a pathway through the wilderness. I will create rivers in the dry wasteland." (Isaiah 43: 19 NLT)

I raised William, as a single mom for 10 years. It was then I met and married Alain, William's step father. William and I have had many talks over the years about the fact that it is love that makes a family, not a blood connection. Ironically, when William's blood type changes over to A+, he will have the same blood type as his step father.

Not only is God answering a long-standing, and very personal prayer of William's, but also He is allowing us to see His Word in action as He changes William's very blood, and creates something new in him.

> *Comment 6: It's so amazing to witness with your own eyes the hand of God at work. It does change you and always for the better. Praying for a speedy recovery. Take care*

> *Comment 7: I want you to know I admire your courage and ability to share all of your thoughts and prayers while going through this ordeal. God is watching over all of you and I especially admire you William because even in the midst of turmoil you have a sense of humor and such a deep faith in your Lord and Savior. When I was reading your post tonight the scripture posted touch my heart so deeply it brought tears to my eyes. I saw that passage in such a different light. Thank You for that. God Bless and you are all always in my prayers.*

January 9
Day -6

William got settled into his hospital room last night about 9:30 p.m. He started full doses of chemo today. He tolerated it pretty well, only needing medicine for nausea twice. He will have three more consecutive days of chemo. I am glad he handled today so well. I know worse days are ahead so I sure am thankful for the better days. He brought a journal with him, and will try to write down how he feels as he goes through this process.

January 10
Day -5

Only five days and counting. William is still holding up, he is walking around (wearing mask and gloves), and meeting some of the other transplant patients. His allergies are beginning to act up and he has started coughing so they are watching closely to make sure no infections rise up. Two more days of chemo to go, then he takes medicine for a few days that will help his body accept the new bone marrow, and lessen the severity of Graft vs. Host Disease (GVHD). GVHD is where the new transplanted cells attack the recipient's body. It can range from mild to severe, so they pre-medicate for it, to help keep it manageable. But GVHD will be a concern for another day; right now the main concern is keeping his allergies in check and preventing infections. He is faithful to wear his mask and gloves when he leaves his room and that is his best source of protection, since his immune system is being destroyed with the chemo. He is fighting hard, and doing great!

January 11
Day -4

One day at a time, we get closer and closer to Day 0. William is still holding on. I talked to William by phone.

He said the chemo makes him pretty nauseated and the night sweats have started back up (another effect of the chemo). He walks several times a day to help keep him active, but he didn't feel much like it this evening. One more day of chemo left!

Tonight - William wrote in his journal, "They have finally removed the IV in my arm after three days. I don't see the purpose in the IV since I have the CVC (chest port). The nausea and abdominal pain is getting much worse now and the nausea meds are starting to lose their potency. I am growing immune to them, or the nausea is getting stronger, either way I can tell I'm about to have some bad days ahead."

Before leaving Houston, I met with the pharmacy and went over the list of post transplant medications William will be taking. In the three months following his transplant, his medications will total just over $100,000! Yes, you read that right! His monthly dose of pills will be over $33,400, and that is with no complications. For whatever medications that are not covered by his Medicaid plan, the pharmacy has programs worked out with the pharmaceutical companies that will help ensure he gets his medicines. That was a huge relief to know they have programs in place to help and that they are filing the paperwork for me. I just need to get the papers to them and they will handle the rest; I can focus on helping William.

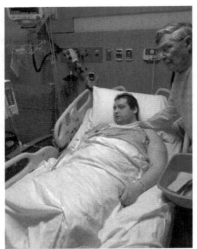

January 12
Day -3

The full-on assault onto William's immune system has begun. Within three days his white cells will be at zero. Between the chemo and the medicine used to bring him to zero, he is struggling now. He has been vomiting since last night, and they have him back in bed instead of up walking around. I knew tougher days were on the horizon, but it doesn't make it any easier. The mom in me just aches as he struggles.

"Therefore do not worry about tomorrow, for tomorrow will worry about itself. Each day has enough trouble of its own." (Matthew 6:34 NIV)

Day -3 Update

Please keep William close to your heart tonight and in your prayers. He is vomiting everything, not able to hold down anything and the medicine isn't really helping. He is also bouncing a fever from 99.3 to 101.3 at the highest. They have taken blood to run cultures to make sure there are no infections, and have started broad spectrum antibiotics as a preventative measure just in case. He is neutropenic at this point and will only get worse in the next few days. Please pray for the fever to leave him and him to be able to hold food on his stomach.

I am not handling this "do not worry" thing very well right now! I am worrying! Doctors are watching very closely and the fever could just be from the medicines. That's not uncommon but there is still a level of concern. I am leaving to return to Houston immediately, and bringing James and Abbey with me. I need to be there with him.

> *Comment 5: I truly ache for William and his family....Its like you just love them all there is....and you pray all there is...and hopefully with Gods help we will follow Williams journey on earth for a long, long time..Thank you God for letting us know him..Amen*

> *Comment 8: I remember with Timothy, he was the same way at this point. It is so hard on them & us too. Love & Prayers!!!!*

> *Comment 10: Always praying for him and am sending more prayers now. Have the docs mentioned anything about TPN? I was on it to make sure i was getting all the vitamins i needed. And it was intravenous. Hang in there William!*

> *Comment 15: I'm completely at a loss of words. I love you and all of your family very dearly. All of you are continually in my prayers.*

> *Comment 18: Praying! My son will be having a BMT in a few weeks so this helps me know what to expect! Praying for William!*

> *Comment 39: Dear Father, most High God, we come humbled to you today, standing in the gap for William and his family. Father, it is at these desperate times of need we cry out to you and Thank You in advance for ministering to William and carrying him to health. Father we declare*

your words, by Jesus's stripes William is healed. Thank you again Father for your goodness and mercies and peace. Amen

January 13
Day -2

William is in contact isolation now. His fever is at 102 this morning and his blood pressure dropped. He is still stable. They do not feel like he needs to go to ICU but if his blood pressure continues to drop, that will be next step. They are running cultures to see if he has any infection or if this is just a reaction to the medication. Again, it's not uncommon to react this way, but there is still a heightened level of concern with his doctors. He is miserable and in pain.

I will probably update a couple times a day for the next few days, simply because I need round the clock prayers for William. Please feel free to share any of the posts I make. I want as many as possible praying for William.

January 14
Day -1

The fevers, low blood pressure, fast heart rate and vomiting continue. The fevers fluctuate between 99.5 up to 103. His blood pressure remains on the low side most of the time and his heart rate is steadfastly high. He isn't able to hold anything down. He just ate a saltine cracker so here in a few minutes that will come back up. I have him drinking Sprite because (sorry this is gross but true), it tastes the same coming up as it does going down!

He has managed to stay out of ICU so far, but they are watching the low blood pressure. The doctor said for us not to panic if it happens, (yeah, right!) as it just means William will get closer monitoring. But so far that hasn't been necessary. All cultures are coming back negative so it appears this is all medication related. This is some horrible stuff they are pumping into him! The goal is to literally obliterate his immune system so he can't fight his new bone marrow when it's introduced. There is no nice way to destroy a body. They do the best they can to try to keep

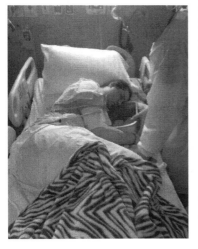

him comfortable but in reality, that's just not possible. He hurts all over, so the best I can do is just hold his hand and remind him it's almost over!

This photo was taken last night. You can see the rash on his shoulder and back area, around the washcloths. We were trying to cool him but his fever was over 103 and the rash was covering his entire body. You can just see how miserable he was!

Comment 26: Goosebumps everywhere! I believe they are more like spirit sparks! I'll be praying from sun up to sundown!

Comment 33: You hang in there..Believe me, I know how you feel. Been there..This May 25th I will celebrate 10 years out..It will all be worth it. Have faith..never give up..and remember, failure is not an option.. I'll be praying for you

January 15
Day 0

The doctor was just in. The bone marrow has not arrived yet, so she is going to try to get an update as to when we can expect it. If it is too late tonight, it will be tomorrow. This happens a lot when the donor is international. I will keep you updated as we learn more.

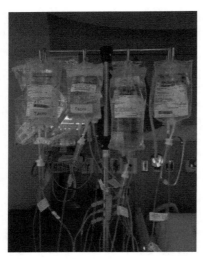

William had a hard night. His fever spiked again. He has chills, rash, swelling, vomiting. The chemo is continuing its assault! The good news is that he is finished with the chemo for now. He will get chemo again after the transplant, but only four small doses spread out over eleven days, and it's not as harsh as this chemo was.

For now, keep praying for William, his donor and for the pilot and the jet that will bring William his new bone marrow. Now is not the time for mechanical issues, bad weather or anything else that could cause a problem!

Day 0 – Update

We have news! The bone marrow will arrive at MDA around midnight so he will get the transplant tomorrow. We don't have a time yet but it's on the way. It's on the way!

William's condition has improved a little today. His fever

is gone. The chills, swelling, pain and neuropathy are being managed with medications - look at all those bags hanging on his IV carousel! The goal is to manage his pain and symptoms through the night and allow him to rest for tomorrow.

"Weeping may tarry through the night, BUT joy comes in the morning." (Psalm 30:5b ESV)

> *Comment 30: That's a breathtaking and deeply moving photograph. So many different types of fluid/medication bags, lines and piggy backs..... that right there is what has to be called: An "Intravenous Pole/Tree of Life".... literally.....*

> *Comment 35: Be strong...so many people praying for you and God has listened...we continue to pray for you so you have the strength to welcome your new day with love from us all*

> *Comment 41: "Come to me, all you who are weary and burdened, and I will give you rest. Take my yoke upon you and learn from me, for I am gentle and humble in heart, and you will find rest for your souls. For my yoke is easy and my burden is light." —Matthew 11:28–30*

January 16
Day 00

Today is a great day! An appointed day! The first thought when I woke up this morning was the verse "I tell you, now is the time of God's favor, now is the day of salvation." (2 Cor. 6:2 NIV)" Today is the day my son will be saved from this horrible cancer!

William is ready. His counts have zeroed out and his marrow is not producing any new blood. What is left of his blood is cycling through his body and dying out. He is ready. The transplant is actually an infusion of the bone marrow, just like a blood transfusion. It will begin between 11:00 a.m. and noon today. The infusion will last about five to seven hours. We learned that his bone marrow was flown from Italy. So we know an origin but not much else. It will be two years before he is allowed to meet his donor, and that is only if they both agree to meet.

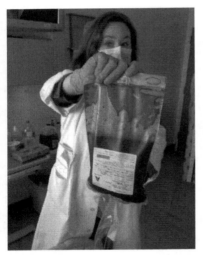

They have started his pre-meds to prepare him. It won't be long now. The doctor called the chaplain to be ready to come bless the new cells. I will post pictures and updates as we progress through the day. Pray, Team William, pray for God's favor on this day and on William!

Update: At 11:28 a.m., new bone marrow flowed into William's body! Day 00, January 16, 2014, Happy Re-Birthday William!

Note: If you would like to see the actual video of the transplant, it can be viewed on William's Facebook page, www.facebook.com/hopeforwilliam.

Comment 4: Like is such a understatement! Thank you for sharing this precious moment with all of us.

Comment 30: Amazing! Bawling like a baby.... Thank you Amy for sharing this Special moment with all us.

Comment 36: Praise our Heavenly Father. I am sitting here weeping for joy and have cold chills on my arms.

Comment 50: OUR GOD IS AN AWESOME! PRAISE GOD FROM WHOM ALL BLESSINGS FLOW.....

January 17
Day +1

I love being on the + side of the countdown now. Today William is receiving two units of his new blood type. The new bone marrow hasn't grafted yet. That will take time so his blood type hasn't changed yet, but the hospital couldn't get any A- blood. He is still very sick from the chemo he took to prepare for the transplant. It is continuing its job of killing his bone marrow, old blood and cancer cells. It will be a hard two weeks as the effects of the chemo peak between days 10-14. He will continue to get blood transfusions as needed until the new bone marrow grafts and starts creating new blood and the chemo wears off. He has to stay in protective isolation until his immune system is able to recover and rebuild.

I still can't believe we are here, on "the other side." It happened - it really happened! Everyone told us the actual transplant would be anticlimactic, but I didn't find that to be so. I watched in complete awe as that bone marrow went into his body, and within an hour I began to see color returning to his skin and his lips. After several hours he was able to sit up, eat a few bites and carry on a conversation. *I watched LIFE return to him!* Once again we watched God's word in action, "The life of all flesh is in the blood."

January 18
Day +2

William is heading downhill! It's expected, but hard to watch. The Busulfan side effects will peak between days 10-14. He will progressively get worse over the next ten days. His entire digestive tract is full of mucus, and ulcers are invading his throat and mouth, and are expected to get much worse before they get better. I asked Dr. Worth and she said it is all normal progression. That is just some awful chemo with one job, to destroy! And it does.

He is spiking fevers and having some fairly violent chills. He feels like hell, and he doesn't talk much. It hurts him. He turned his phone off and put it away so if you call or text him, please understand that he is probably not going to respond for several days. He isn't ignoring anyone; he is just too sick right now.

He only had one unit of blood yesterday because of his fever and chills. They had to give him A+ because they could not get A- or O. They ran labs and it was safe to give him the A+ because that was his donor's type, but it shows how desperately low the blood supply is. Please, please, please if you can give blood - do it. If you are in the Houston area, come to MDA. If you are in a reasonable driving distance, load the car, van or fill a bus and come donate. If you aren't near Houston, then donate locally. I am sure the holidays and now the flu outbreak has taken a devastating toll on the blood supply everywhere. One whole blood donation is divided out and will save up to three lives. Platelets are also critically low. It is far better for a patient to receive a single donor bag of platelets than a multiple donor bag.

The life of all flesh is in the blood. These patients need you, so they can live.

January 19
Day +3

That chemo was some bad stuff! I noticed William's feet are turning black and the doctor said he was going to lose one toenail for sure, possibly more. The skin on his tongue is peeling off. The whites of his eyes are bloody, caused by low platelets. He can't blow his nose or he will get a nose-bleed that will last for hours. These are only a part of the side effects, there are more. This is not for the squeamish!

Even still, he managed to get out of bed and take a walk. It's important to fight through the pain and keep your muscles active. Today he received a unit of platelets, and will continue to get them regularly until his counts begin to recover, in about two weeks. He will need blood again; his hemoglobin level is very low. He will be using a lot of blood products in the next few weeks.

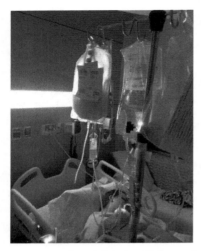

January 20
Day +4

I knew this process was going to be hard, but I was not prepared for just how hard. I sat on the couch in William's room just crying, wishing the vicious assault on his body would stop! He woke up vomiting blood. The whites of his eyes are continuing to fill with blood. Dr. Worth said it is all from his low platelet count; it is near 0 right now.

This bag of yellow liquid is a bag of platelets...liquid gold, liquid LIFE! This bag will keep him from bleeding out. He will need daily bags, sometimes multiple bags a day.

He can't speak from the pain in his mouth and throat so we are communicating through a series of grunts, pointing and hand signals. To try to keep him comfortable they are setting him up on a PCA pump (morphine pump) and keeping him on cough syrup to limit the coughing and vomiting. I am trying to prepare myself for the fact it will actually get worse before it gets better, but there is no real way to prepare for this! The chemo effects peak at days 10-14, so my only consolation is that we are getting closer to relief, one day at a time. We need those prayers for each and every day.

Thank you to everyone who is holding William up in prayer right now, and ministering to me as well. I think of the story in the Bible when the people of Israel went to battle and Moses told Joshua he would stand on the hill, holding the staff of God. As long Moses held up the staff, the Israelites had the advantage. But Moses grew weary and he could no longer bear the weight and burden of holding the staff up so Aaron and Hur helped Moses. He sat on a stone while Aaron and Hur stood on either side of him, holding his arms steady until sunset, and victory. You are our Aaron and Hur right now, holding us up when we aren't able to in our own strength.

> *Comment 9: I have been sick & off Facebook for a couple days. I'm not surprised to see this post, as I turned so ill after my transplant, receiving many transfusion. Just outright feeling awful! Accepting the doctors saying "this is where you should be: we expect this.." Is HARD! I promise I was there, just 7 short months ago...it's hard but worth every bit of the fight. Continued prayers for William & family!*

> *Comment 14: (((HUGS))) There is no way to be prepared for it. I say over and over that those were the worst days of my life watching Hannah go through that. I can only imagine how it felt for her. Hang in there!!*

> *Comment 20: Unending prayers for William are being sent to our gracious Heavenly Father. May The Lord bless you and keep you, make His face shine upon you, and give you peace.*

January 21
Day +5

Today William had two units of blood and more platelets. One unit was of his current blood type, A- and the second one was A+, which is what his blood will become after the grafting process. He doesn't seem to react to the new blood type, which surprises me since he hasn't started grafting yet. They check his blood type every morning and it is still A-. His eyes are still bloody, now both eyes are about 50% white and 50% bloody. The eyes kind of freak him out a little bit. He said he looks like he has been in a fight.

The doctor more than doubled his pain meds and it seemed to help him. He has been more alert today and is able to move around more. Tomorrow's goal will be to take another walk, no matter how bad it hurts.

His white cells increased from 0 to .2 and while this doesn't seem like something to celebrate, it actually is. It means his body is trying to recover from the chemo. The recovery is a very slow process but anything in the right direction is a victory. We still have several days left till we get past the peak effects of the chemo, but we will just have to take it one day at a time.

One thing that puzzles me, if not concerns me is that his hair hasn't fallen out. It always happens with transplants, but his hasn't even started thinning. Anyone with transplant experience have any advice on this?

> *Comment 2: his hair will fall out on day 11, (I predict)..and it won't thin..he will be in the shower and poof, will come out bald..(I predict)..at least that is how it went for me, and I had the same protocol..I am thinking about each and every day, reliving, to some extent, my transplant, almost 10 years ago..you are doing well..glad to hear that his white count is beginning to recover. Once it does, your pain will go away, the sores will clear up and then you will be able to go into PT to regain your*

strength..that is not far away..there is a teeny tiny light beginning to shine..

Comment 3: I still had some hair when you look at my transplant day. I lost what I had again around day 10 to day 15. Praying for y'all and big hugs. All is the right direction.

Comment 11: Darling: he HAS been in a fight. We know it and support him and are grateful for any recovery!

Comment 20: My hair didn't fall out until about 2 weeks after transplant..

January 22
Day +6

Amp up those prayers, William is having a traumatic day! He had a very hard night, and this morning while trying to take his meds, he began to vomit pretty violently. He said it was like swallowing a razor, and then he felt a weird pressure deep in his throat, then a pulling, tearing, "uncorking" sensation. He threw up the entire lining of his esophagus in one "blob." He immediately went into shock, of course.

The nurse was in the room while it happened and I am very grateful. She was able to help calm him and explain that this can happen. Once his white cells recover the body will heal itself and rebuild the esophageal lining. Until then, his medications will be switched to IV form. He isn't able to eat or drink anything. He can't speak so he writes messages and I am teaching him some simple sign language to help us communicate better. If he can't eat at all they will give him IV nutrition, which is common and expected.

He did take a walk this morning, even after the trauma and I expect another lap around the nurse station later today.

We are getting into the thick of it so please keep him uplifted in prayer over the next several days.

January 23
Day +7

When I went to bed last night William had hair. When I woke up he was nearly totally bald. Overnight! It was unbelievable! He said he couldn't sleep and his hair just came out in his hands all night. He still hasn't been able to eat or drink anything at all, but they are monitoring his labs to see when they need to start IV nutrition. He had more platelets today and managed to take another walk. I can't even begin to imagine the pain he is in, and I am so proud of him for fighting through. He wrote in his journal that he is in incredible pain all over his body. His throat hurts to even breathe. He feels like thousands of wasps are stinging him all at once through his feet and hands. He is terrified beyond belief.

January 24
Day +8

I heard the phrase "you would be surprised what you can live through" in a movie years ago...yep!

I mentioned before the skin on William's tongue is coming off. Last night he lost a little too much skin and his mouth was openly bleeding. The on-call doctor ordered some platelets immediately to help stop the bleeding. Today he

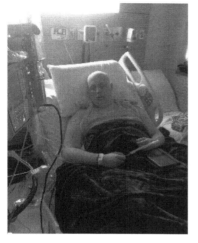

is getting two units of blood. The medications that help prevent reactions to blood transfusions make him sleep, which is good! He needs the deep sleep.

His white cells are at 0. Once they begin to recover, so will he. He is getting Neupogen shots to help that. He still hasn't been able to eat or drink anything at all. His weight is dropping pretty fast. At first he gained weight even though he was barely eating, but it was just water weight from all the fluids they are pumping into him. His doctor is watching labs and said IV nutrition will probably start tomorrow. The benchmark they look for is low, but not quite low enough yet.

After the first unit of blood we will try to get a lap around the nurses' station, before second unit arrives. Through it all, he remains in good spirits and doesn't grumble or complain. He said this transplant better work, cause he isn't doing this a second time! Again, a little humor laced with a smidgen of truth.

January 25
Day +9

Today we made "ice mittens" for William. Let me explain,

neuropathy continues to be a problem with his hands and feet. This is caused by the chemo and will last for several months after discharge, but will eventually go away (we hope). It was being controlled by medication but since he can't swallow his pills, and there is no IV substitution, he just has to suffer through it. The skin on his hands and feet have turned deep purplish to black and is burning hot, itches, and feels like razors slashing at it when you touch it. So we filled some surgical gloves with ice, tied them in a knot, sealed them in ziploc baggies and shoved that into a sock. He has them for both hands and feet. It seems to be helping to relieve some of the pain.

It has been three days since William threw up the lining of his esophagus and he has not been able to eat or drink anything since. Not even a teaspoon of water, he tried yesterday and it was disastrous! With that, I have a very specific prayer request. Please ask God to heal his throat! With his throat healed he could eat and drink again and take the medication he needs for his neuropathy.

> *Comment 16: I know it's not right. But I have a hard time trying to imagine Will's current condition without starting to cry.. Tell him he's my best friend in the world and I wish I could be there beside him. But deep down I know he can fight this, since he told me himself and Will is too honest to lie to me. I'm still trying to open my heart to God for Will, but I've found it's not the easiest thing in the world when you aren't blessed with the gift of faith.. But I'm trying regardless! Hopefully God can still hear me..*

> *Comment 28: Praying. Kyle, faith isn't a gift. It's a choice. To believe...or not. It's learned, in baby steps. But God can always hear you. Always. You*

just have to surrender yourself to hear him back. And that's the catch, isn't it? Giving up yourself to become who God wants you to be. Thankfully, he likes us as we are, at our core. He made us, after all. So it's not as scary as we make it out to be. You just have to choose who you will serve. God? Or You. It's something we all struggle with. You aren't alone in that. *hugs*

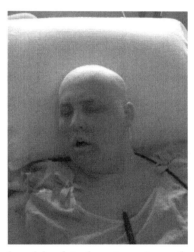

January 26
Day +10

William is very weak today, and very pale. He is in and out sleep. He has not eaten in four days. His hemoglobin is low and platelets are very low. The shortage of platelets has reached a critical level and the hospital has to ration them out. Yesterday a patient's platelet level had to be at 20 in order to get an infusion, today they had to lower that to 15. William was at 18 at 5:00 a.m. With both platelet and hemoglobin levels so low, I requested (demanded, rather) they retest him at 4:00 this afternoon. By then his levels should drop low enough to qualify for an infusion. His white cells are still at zero. I know we are in the darkest days right now. We are all waiting with baited breath for him to turn around. His white cells need to recover, his throat needs to heal.

"The Lord will fight for you, you need only be still." Thank you to the one who sent me that verse!

January 27
Day +11

Not much new news to report. White cells still at zero, William's hemoglobin was low today so he is getting two units of blood and one of platelets. Any day now his white cells should begin to recover. That's our #1 prayer right now. Once that happens, his throat will heal.

He has a suction tube in his mouth, like the one dentists use, to suck the mucus, saliva and blood from his mouth and throat since he can't swallow anything. There is still so much blood in his mucus! He fills the container every day, and it's about 6 cups of just blood and mucus. Luckily, we haven't had any new surprises in the last day or two. It's just waiting and watching the lab reports right now. Come on white blood cells!

> *Comment 6: The scripture just came to mind..Those who wait upon the Lord SHALL renew their strength..They SHALL mount upon wings as eagles...they SHALL run and not be weary....this waiting is hard I know so well...But necessary...that cell will kick in and all this will be behind you...I believe that will all my heart, soul and being and spirit...I wish I could just wrap my arms around all of you and hold you and cry and laugh with you...Joy comes in the morning sweet family..*

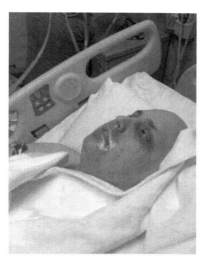

January 28
Day +12

Today William will receive more blood and platelets. He still cannot swallow anything so we are at day 6 with no food or water and walking is nearly impossible with the neuropathy in his feet. He shakes so violently from the pain when he tries to stand up!

Death is near my son. I can smell him; I can feel him lingering in the room with us, just waiting for William to give up fighting. If I could fight for him I would, if I could give him my strength, I would. I just sat next to William, as he was going in and out of consciousness, and whispered in his ear to keep fighting, don't give up! Over and over I reminded him the worst is almost over, just don't give up now. I begged God not to take him from me. I'm not ready to say good-bye! I asked God to reach down and touch him, to touch him with His physical hand so William could feel Him, and give William comfort and strength and help him fight. Just please don't take him from me!

> *Comment 1: HOPE*
> *Hold*
> *On*
> *Pain*
> *Ends*

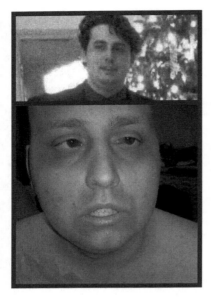

January 29
Day +13

Take a long hard look at this picture. The top picture was taken Christmas Day 2012, just six months before William was diagnosed. The bottom picture was taken yesterday. THIS is what cancer looks like, THIS is what leukemia does!

A friend sent me Psalm 23 this morning, and it says "yea, though I walk through the valley of the shadow of death, I will fear no evil; for thou art with me; thy rod and thy staff, they comfort me." William is in the valley, but he knows his Lord and he told me the other night he isn't afraid, no matter what. He believes, as do I, that he will beat this. Today his white cells were at .1 but they didn't drop, so it's good. He is in the valley, but he is coming through!

> Comment 13: *He is in the valley but praise God he has started up the mountain and when he gets to the top there will be a lot of people shouting and praising God for Williams complete healing. Leukemia is horrible for anyone to have but when you get through it you are stronger than you have ever been. God Bless both of you*

> Comment 40: *William is just walking through the valley, not staying there! Stay strong William! The Lord is fighting with you!*

Comment 60: I see a beautiful young man in both pictures...just one with a harder battle than the other...prayers from the bottom of my heart...

January 30
Day +14

William was able to take a sip of water today! His first in 8 days! It hurt like... well... you know, but he managed to get it down. This is a huge step in recovery! I am thrilled! I have said it before; we celebrate EVERY victory, no matter how big or small! I also noticed last night William was forcing himself to stand, even though the neuropathy in his feet makes it nearly impossible. He is pushing himself to his limits, and that means he is feeling stronger. It means he is healing and recovering! His voice is trying to come back. He is getting stronger, little by little. His white cells have camped out at 0.1 but I can see outward expressions of inside strengthening so I am encouraged. Today he received two more units of blood and one of platelets. These daily transfusions of blood products will only help to make him stronger.

Today, I headed back home for a few days so I can spend time with my husband and my younger two kids (ages three and five), and take care of household stuff. Mom and Dad are going to take care of William in my absence. It is very hard not being there! This has been an ongoing struggle for me, to find the balance of my time for all my kids. My little ones are too young to be at the hospital, and to be honest if it were not for my parents and my husband, I could never do this. Mom and Dad take care of my little ones while I am with William and they take care of William while I am with my little ones. And Alain, my husband, makes it possible for me to just focus on being "mom" wherever I am. I am eternally grateful!

January 31
Day +15

It has been nine days with no measurable water and no food at all. William said he wasn't able to drink anything today so he just swallowed a little spit to test his throat. His white cells are still at 0.1 and just haven't budged in days. We really need to pray those white cells get in there and heal his throat so he can finally eat and drink and actually get some nutrients to his body. The doctors do not want to give him TPN (IV nutrition) because it is hard on the liver, and his liver levels are already elevated.

William said he just feels tired today, which is understandable. The chemo continues to attack him through his skin and the neuropathy in his hands and feet. William is still forcing himself to stand and take steps around his room, no matter how bad it hurts. The throat healing is key! Once he can swallow again, he can get the neuropathy medicine in liquid form and can get some relief and some much needed nutrients to his body.

Please just pray for healing and endurance; he really needs it.

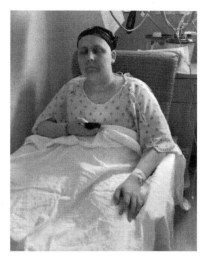

February 1
Day +16

White cell count is 0.2 today! William continues to amaze me with his strength! He sat in the chair today and so far he has drunk 8 ounces of water. It is the first measurable amount of ANYTHING in 10 days. He said he will try to drink a little more later. What a warrior!

Comment 2: The fight this man has is indescribable! God continue to be with him!

Comment 34: Way to go William! You do the possible and let God do the impossible..Praising God for the 0.2 and asking for a continuous raise in WBC and for your complete healing. Every second of every day is a miracle. Keep praising Him!!!

February 2
Day +17

Still no food, only water. It has been 11 days with nothing to eat. I am hoping tomorrow William will be able to drink a Boost or an Ensure, just anything with some nutritional value. He is now able to take some of his medicines in a liquid form and he said his throat feels a little better today.

His hemoglobin counts seem to be holding steady but he is still getting daily platelets. His doctors were hoping for higher white cell counts but are very encouraged that he hasn't had any fever or infections. These are good signs! He is still pushing himself past the pain to stand and take short walks around his room. He is even joking a little tonight and trying to smile! All great signs of recovery...now those white cells just need to catch up.

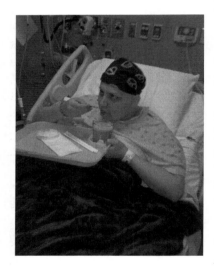

Day 17 update-

Finally! He is "eating" something, technically he is drinking, but still! It's a Boost shake, but it's the first bit of food in 11 days. I am a very happy Mama right now!

Comment 2: GOD BLESS U. ARE SO STRONG U WILL WIN DAMN CANCER SUCKS! LOL AND MANY PRAYERS!!!! AMEN

Comment 57: Yes, GOD IS GREAT! I lost from 187 to 160. 30 days without almost any food or drink! Slept almost the entire time.

February 3
Day +18

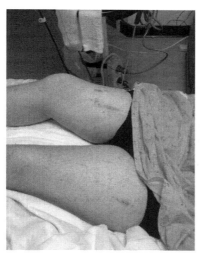

William's white cells are 0.3! They need to get to 0.5 before we will know if he is grafting, hopefully by the end of the week. He is doing fine with the liquid diet, not quite ready to introduce solid food yet, maybe next week. For now the nutritionist is happy with the Boost. William has slept most of the day. He was itching like crazy and they gave him a healthy dose of Benedryl. He has to be careful scratching, the low platelets cause him to get these claw marks and they will bleed with just a little scratching. If the platelets get too low, he can't stop bleeding so they watch that very closely.

I talked to the doctor on the phone today, and he is very pleased with William's progress. He was very encouraged, as am I. William and I talked for quite some time on the phone this morning too, and he is sounding more like his normal self. I think it is safe to say he finally turned the corner and is now headed toward recovery!

February 4
Day +19

William received two units of blood and another unit of platelets today. He has been itchy and nauseated, and we were wondering if that was GVHD (Graft vs. Host Disease) but the doctor said not yet. First the donor cells will make white blood cells, then red, then platelets. Then the donor cells will mature and kill any of William's remaining cells, including any residual leukemia cells. That's when the GVHD will show up. It can attack the skin, liver or other organs. They want to see *some* GVHD because it means the new cells are doing what they are supposed to do, but we need to start praying for a mild case of GVHD. Eventually the new blood will take over his marrow completely and the new blood system will live in harmony with the rest of his body. The white blood cells reaching 0.5 is key, today he is still at 0.3 and holding. Praying for 0.4 tomorrow and some relief from the nausea and other effects from the chemo he took nearly three weeks ago. In his journal, William wrote that one of the side effects of the Neupogen shots is intense bone pain. He said it feels like his legs are in a wood splitter. He said he feels like he did in the days before his diagnosis.

February 5
Day +20

Are you ready for it?
White cells aren't 0.4,
they aren't 0.5...
as of this morning William's white cells are 1.1!

The doctor said he could start seeing GVHD signs at any time now. That means HE IS GRAFTING! The donor cells are taking over! His skin is still in the process of chafing off and rebuilding from the chemo he received pre-transplant (that is what causes the dark brown/black splotches on him). Now we need to look for skin GVHD and they will monitor closely for internal GVHD attacking his organs. His doctor says right now his number one goal is for William to get calories. He doesn't care how he gets them; he just needs to get more calories.

William wasn't in the mood to get his picture taken today, so we are going to respect that request. While we were all doing the victory dance when we got the news, he said he didn't feel very victorious. He feels like crap!

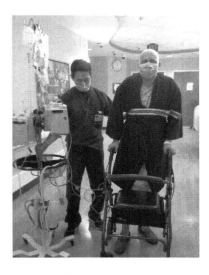

February 6
Day +21

Three weeks! William's white cells are at 2.2! His absolute neutrophil count (ANC) is 1.61. When the ANC is above .5 for three consecutive days they will stop the Neupogen shots in the stomach. Then his white cells will drop in half. Once the white cells start increasing after that drop, it means the new marrow is working and producing new blood.

Now William NEEDS to eat! He isn't even getting 300 calories a day, and his doctor said he has got to get more calories. Plus he is having severe bone pain. This could be from the Neupogen shots or his marrow trying to produce blood, as it causes the bones to swell. Either way, it is very painful. But still he walks. God is amazing! Look at William. He is up, he is ALIVE! I am still processing all of this. It's a lot to take in.

It was eight months ago today that he was taken to the hospital, and this journey began. There were times of crushing pain and sorrow when I didn't know if he would survive, days when I would replay the video of him playing his guitar over and over wondering if it would be last time I heard him play, days when I wondered if I would be strong enough if I had to plan his funeral - terrible days! But there were also days when I could hear God promising me William would live, days where only my faith allowed me to keep going, to keep hoping, to keep believing, and some days just to keep breathing.

I wish I could say I never questioned God, but that's just not true. I wanted to never doubt but there were days when I did. But every time I would doubt I would see the verse "is anything too wonderful for The Lord?" It would come in emails, Facebook posts, it was everywhere. It was God reminding me to keep my eyes on Him and not on circumstances. He was whispering "when you can't trace My hand, trust My heart." Yes, it would have been easier if the clouds would have parted and God would have written in the sky, "Hey Amy, I got this!" But that's not really how faith works is it?

I have said before that I am not strong enough to handle this, and I am not - not on my own. But I gather strength from reading God's Word and looking back on where He has seen us through. I gain strength from you. Your prayers and words of encouragement help me tremendously. I also gain strength from William. Not only does he fight this with grace that most people will never see, but also he doesn't question or resent God. He just trusts and believes that no matter what happens to him, it is God's will, and he is a winner either way, and THAT my friends is faith in action!

Comment 9: Amazing! Keep fighting William! Amy I am so thankful for your daily updates. You are so strong, whether you feel it or not. You are all covered up in prayer from all over!

Comment 17: Yeah! Go William! Amy you have done a wonderful job raising this fine young man!!! What a fighter!!

Comment 23: Amy each time I read your post tears fill my eyes because I have been where you are. Taking one-day at a time. I feel like I have known you my whole life. I told Katie I wish I could meet you and William. I look for your post everyday and I keep checking till you post. There was times I didn't think I was going to make it watching Katie be so sick she couldn't hold her head up but God always filled me with strength. There was a few times I didn't think Katie was going to make it through it but God always sent me something or someone to let me know to just trust him that he had this just trust. It will be five years April 21st when our journey start but praise God Katie gets better and better. I guess the reason I feel so close to you is William is the same age Katie was when she got diagnosed. God Bless both of you and the rest of your family.

Comment 29: My daughter was diagnosed with leukaemia in October 2012. She was 17 months old. She had a bone marrow transplant in March 2013. She has been in remission for 11 months now. Transplant is so hard and there are a lot of dark days. But it saved her life. It was the best gift she could've been given. I pray for William every day that he recovers quickly and will soon be free of this horrible disease.

Comment 33: I don't know you William but am keeping up with your story. I don't have to tell you that God is AMAZING because you already know that. Keep up the great work and be sure to eat. Prayers to you and you mom for strength.

Comment 34: Such an inspiration! God is working through you and William to encourage everyone who reads your post to trust in God no matter the circumstances. That is the only peace we can have in times of turmoil. William continues to be in my prayers. Praying for strength, relief, appetite and a full recovery. God bless you all.

Comment 40: I really don't know you either, but don't give up on having faith in God! Pray and fight for your life!' I just know in my heart you will make it. God answers prayers in mysterious ways! Win this one William.

Comment 55: You don't know me. And yet, I know that every word you say is the truth. It's odd, it's is? How such utter pain, sadness, even fear, can also exist in your heart where the peace that comes from knowing that we do not walk alone and that all will be well also dwells. Thank you for sharing your story. Keep strong knowing that prayers are yours and William's from unknown people like me.

Comment 60: Amy, you're words seared my soul! Your faith, the strength you've gained through our Lord has filled me with a renewed hope and joy! I stand with you and trust God. He is faithful to complete the work He has begun. Thank you for sharing such intimate and heartfelt thoughts. God's blessings are upon you and William.

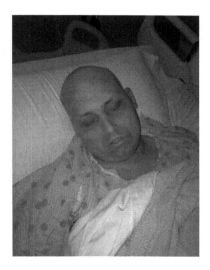

February 7
Day +22

Yesterday was great, today not so much. William continues to hurt everywhere. His nurse really wanted him to take his meds in pill form and he promptly vomited them back up. He is staying on IV meds until his throat has more time to heal. He is coughing a lot more, and having some symptoms and pains that could be indicative to GVHD of the gut. The best way to diagnose it is to do a biopsy so that's on tap for next week. His skin is continuing to turn black and peel off. It's just a rough phase right now!

But there is good news too. His white cells and ANC are still good, and the best news is that he had his first hot meal today. He had about half a bowl of very brothy chicken and rice. Then, with a full belly, he promptly fell into a peaceful deep sleep.

February 8
Day +23

Today has been a bit of a setback. William has started vomiting again, and as of this evening he hasn't been able to eat. My goal for now is just to get him eating again, even tiny bits every hour is better than nothing. He has also tested positive for VRE, an infection that is common in transplant patients, so that is being watched and closely monitored. His skin continues to turn black and peel off. He was washing his hands and looked in the mirror and told me he looks like a corpse. It really bothers him to look this way! I am hoping for a more positive day tomorrow.

I also want to ask you all to keep a special family in your prayers. Yesterday evening another warrior was called to Heaven. Zach was nine years old, and had AML. He had his transplant two days ahead of William. He was on his THIRD transplant and died from a complication. I can't even begin to imagine the crushing pain his family is going through. Sometimes there just are no words.

> *Comment 3: Sorry William's day wasn't better. I am just glad to see him hanging in there; tell him it doesn't matter to us how he looks, it matters to us how he's doing and how he's holding up as he fights this battle. Any time I see him awake, reading, standing, etc., he looks handsome to me! What a fighter!*

> *Comment 19: William you are strong, you are handsome-inside & out. Love U*

> *Comment 43: I was devastated to hear of Zach 's passing!! There are no words capable of expressing our feelings of sorrow and regret !!*

Prayers for his family that GOD will sustain them through this time !! He fought a long and hard fight and was very courageous ! William will fight through this as he has all along! I love you young man!!

Comment 61: stay strong William! We all know you will be dressing better than everyone else and looking handsome before you know it! Thinking of you and your family tonight and looking forward to a fabulous recovery in the coming week!

Comment 90: I hated the mirrors during transplant..I asked the nurses to cover them! Still praying you got this William!

Comment 94: We are praying for both William and Zach's family. Tell William to hang in there. I felt the same way about how I looked--it stinks-- but it is only for a season.

Comment 100: You tell him, that I don't think he looks like a corpse, but more like an inspiration to me. An inspiration to never give up and never take anything for granted. I have been watching your posts and he is a hero along with all of you that are guiding him and holding his hand everyday. Prayers, prayers, prayers continue for you all.

Comment 105: William looks like a fighter not a corpse. I see a handsome young man with a heart of gold who is fighting his way back to health!! You ROCK in my book William. I follow Zach & I'm heartbroken about him. He is now with Adain (80) & they are no longer suffering.

God Bless William, you & your whole family.
Thanks for keeping us posted.

February 9
Day +24

Only victories today, small ones, but we are taking everything we can get. This morning William was able to eat two small Italian Ice cups and one Popsicle. We managed to get the nausea under better control, and he has not thrown up at all today. He has been able to sip a little water too. I had a long, slightly forceful, talk with his doctor and we have agreed that William will stay on IV and liquid medications until William feels his throat is well enough to swallow pills. And they are to stop pestering him to take the pills! When he is ready, he will do it, but they need to let him take the lead here. Even water is still difficult to swallow, but I keep pushing him to take sips of something, anything every hour. He has been knocked out since he got his pre-meds for his platelets this afternoon.

Tomorrow they are planning to do an endoscopy and a biopsy of his upper GI tract to confirm or rule out GVHD of the gut. He is showing some symptoms of it, but it could be something else too, so they need to know for sure so he can be treated correctly and not let anything get "out of hand." Not sure when we will have those results but we will be waiting anxiously.

February 11
Day +26

Yesterday was one of "those" days, and I didn't update because no matter what or how I typed it, my frustrations were coming through. It was a hard day for William, both physically and emotionally. He is tired of hospitals and hospital beds and nurses and tubes attaching him to IV poles. He is just sick and tired of being sick and tired. Yesterday there was a major miscommunication between a nurse and the on-call evening doctor that caused a big problem with William's medication. William was writhing in pain with tears rolling down his cheeks, and the doctor just wasn't doing anything about it. I finally had to have a "Come to Jesus" talk with the doctor to get something done. His regular doctor came in this morning and we discussed the issue last night. He quickly realized the mistake and made sure it was fixed. I feel much better after talking with him, and having his assurances that it will not happen again.

Now, on to better things. William has been eating a little bit. So far mac-n-cheese and Italian Ice is it, but tonight we are going to try mashed potatoes too. He has had to really struggle to keep it down but so far has done well. He is still a long way from where his doctor wants him to be, but he is getting there. The pre-transplant chemo has altered his taste buds which is another reason eating is hard. Nothing tastes good.

The results from the biopsy should be in tomorrow. But the visual results from the endoscopy look good. William's esophagus and stomach look like they're healing nicely. His white cells and neutrophil counts are doing well. He took a walk today. Now the goals are longer walks and eating more. His doctor is encouraged with his progress and hopes if it continues that he can be discharged in a couple of weeks. He still has to stay in Houston for daily blood checks and follow up appointments for a few months, but at least everything is moving in the right direction.

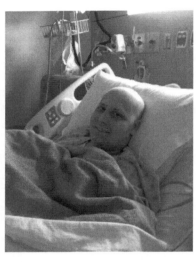

February 12
Day +27

He smiles! Last night William decided to take another walk at 10:30 p.m. So there we were strolling through the hallways while he sings "Mr. Sandman."

Here is something interesting too, he is having strange dreams. He is dreaming of people whom he doesn't know. They are like "ghost images" and they talk but he can't hear them. We did a little reading and we found this is a common phenomenon with blood recipients and transplant patients. They report feeling like someone is "with them" and they have strange dreams and thoughts that are not their own. William said that with the people in his dreams, he feels like he should know them but he doesn't. He also sees a lot of cobblestone and curvy, skinny walkways. A lot of tan color. Very interesting...*the life of all flesh is in the blood.*

He is eating some beef ravioli tonight. Here's to hoping it stays down.

February 13
Day +28

Not too many smiles today! William hasn't felt well all day. He is getting his second unit of blood now. He obviously needs it. He is so pale, especially his lips. He has been fighting nausea all day and the biopsy did confirm GVHD of the gut. That isn't the news we were hoping for but now that we know, we can get a jump on treating it so it doesn't get out of control.

William will see a team of GVHD specialists to help him. He will also have bone marrow biopsy in the next few days. They will be looking to see if grafting has started and to what degree his new marrow is producing, and they will be looking for leukemia. This really worried William. Just the thought that this may not have worked is weighing pretty heavy on him. The doctor and I reminded him that this test is standard and does not indicate his leukemia is back, but it is the only way to know for sure. So, we need a lot of prayers for grafting, NO LEUKEMIA CELLS, to be able to switch to pill-form medicines and continued strength to get up and keep walking.

> Comment 2: Remember, dear friend, that a little GVHD is a good thing ~ it helps fight off any remaining Leukemia cells. Hoping William feels better soon. This picture brings back many memories ~ #CureLeukemia

> Comment 20: I'm so sorry to hear that this day was not a good one. As far as the biopsy goes, it is not uncommon for them to do additional ones. I had GVHD of the gut, also. I know how incredibly frustrating it is. There are good days, and there

are bad days...but gradually the good ones start to outnumber the bad. Don't get yourself down, even if you have a setback. You've got a lot of people in your corner, praying for you. I hope tomorrow is better, William.

Comment 37: Hold on William. Stay strong. Dear God in Heaven, please wrap your loving arms around William and give him peace and comfort. Amen.

Comment 40: As a leukemia survivor and transplant recipient, I know all too well what William is going through. This is by far the hardest part because you have no immune system and you feel awful...and you don't know if your new marrow has "taken" or not. So my words to William are the same words one of my nurses said to me when I was in this stage of treatment - "this will NOT last...it WILL get better". Just hang on and have faith that better times are just around the corner. I am almost 2 years post-BMT and I'm healthy and feeling great. I'm proof of how successful BMT's can be. You'll get there too - I will pray for that.

February 14
Day +29

Happy Valentine's Day! More biopsy results came in today, and again confirmed that William has GVHD of the gut. They tested three separate areas and all three are positive. It is level 1 now, which is good. Level 4 is bad. The treatment plan is to start IV steroids until he can swallow pills again. Then there is a pill-form steroid, Budesonide, that has less negative side effects. Right now he is back to vomiting up everything, so he has quit eating again. The steroids should increase his appetite and almost "force" him to eat, which would not be a bad thing. He just feels awful, but Dr. P says we should see results quickly so he should be feeling better very soon. I am so ready to see that smile again.

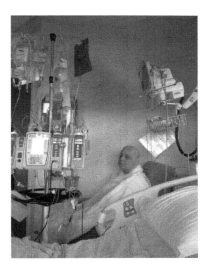

February 15
Day +30

What a milestone - 30 days! Today William was able to eat about 25% of an omelet and keep it down. The steroids seem to be helping the nausea so we are back on track. He is sitting in the chair today watching the History Channel. He is not quite up to walking yet, but just getting up and out of bed is good. Now he needs to re-train his throat to swallow pills again, so that's another goal for him. He may not feel very amazing right now, but he sure is in my eyes.

February 16
Day +31

Wahooooo! The IV steroids have kicked in and went straight for the appetite! William had an omelet for breakfast, salmon *and* BBQ for lunch with flan for dessert.

So far everything is staying down. Since it has been so long since he has eaten anything remotely normal, I was actually worried he would make himself sick. He said tomorrow he is going to attempt to take the steroid pill. Another huge step for him.

The damaged skin on his hands is peeling off now. He still has a lot of black, blotchy, burned patches of skin left to peel off. This is still the aftermath of the chemo he got pre-transplant (over 32 days ago). Even with the peeling skin, I have noticed he is looking so much better.

> *Comment 5: Yay! So happy. Progress. Day by Day. What a fighter! Prayers and Big Hugs to you both!*

> *Comment 47: Such happy news! Steroids...keep the appetite happy!!!!!!! Love U William!*

> *Comment 53: Eat it all, kid! Love you millions!!!*

February 17
Day +32

William has been asleep all day. In fact it was very difficult to wake him up long enough for him to take his liquid medications. There was no way I could get him to try the steroid pill, he simply could not stay awake long enough. This pill is critical to helping his GVHD! We really need "all hands on deck" praying that he can get this pill swallowed. He is showing some possible symptoms of GVHD in the lower gut as well. This is not good news and this steroid pill will help him, but not if he can't take it. Please just pray he can get this pill down. I am open to suggestions, if anyone has ideas on how to make it go down easier. Already asked, and we cannot crush it. It needs to be swallowed whole so it can dissolve in the right place. Ideas?

Comment 2: I used to put mine in applesauce. It was a lot easier to get the pills down. Especially when you have to take so many.

Comment 3: Could he take it with some pudding? Anything to help it slide down easier

Comment 4: Maybe try swallowing with yogurt. It would coat it and help it go down easier.

Comment 5: Put it in some cheese- works for my pups not to make light of a very serious situation. Hope he can get it taken soon. I donated a double platelet this morning. Thought about you guys the whole time!

Comment 6: Ice cream or jello!

Comment 7: We used gel capsule. You can order them online, they even have flavored ones.

Comment 10: ICE CREAM! Pleeeease take your meds!!! We are ALL pulling & praying for you!!!!

Comment 11: I am sorry to hear he can't swallow his steroid pill. I wish I could think of something that would work. I thank God Katie didn't have it in her stomach. She lost fifty pounds because of the mucusitis. She couldn't eat for over three weeks. We tried everything you could possible try. Have they gave him that magic mouth wash it is suppose to numb the throat. Bless his heart I pray God touches his stomach and throat so he can start getting back to where he can eat and drink. Tell him to hang in there. Are you doing okay Amy ? I will continue to pray for both of you. God Bless

Comment 13: Try something cold or inside a noodle, and have him hold his head up and stretch his neck. Think of a baby bird!

February 18
Day +33

Nothing but praises! William was able to swallow the pill and he took a walk without using his walker! He ate well and had no vomiting. Oh, what a great day, what a great day!

He had his bone marrow biopsy this morning, so now we wait for the results. I am just waiting to hear the words *"cancer free, no leukemia cells."* Oh God, how I want to hear those words!

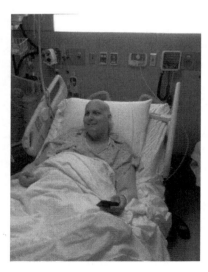

February 19
Day +34

William now has *four* medications in pill form, and he asked his nurse to go ahead and switch one more from liquid to pill. The much needed steroid pill is working wonders with his GVHD, so there is incredible overall improvement.

William and Dr. P have set a goal for William to be discharged next week. He still has to stay within twenty minutes of the hospital for another couple months, so he can't go home yet. But we are getting closer.

Right now we are listening to 80's music on the phones and laughing, watching *Cowboys & Aliens* and waiting on our milkshakes.

February 21
Day +36

I drove home for my niece's wedding this weekend and to spend time with my other little kiddos and hubby. It's hard being one mom in two places. My parents are taking good care of William in my absence, though.

Today was another good day. William is eating well and his nausea is pretty well controlled. He is on target to be released to the apartment next week. It will still be a few months before he can actually make the trip home, and he will be in contact isolation for a while yet.

Now for the best news...preliminary reports from the bone marrow biopsy have come in. According to the doctor, "It looks good, real good!" We won't have full results yet on blast percentage or engraftment for several weeks, but for now, at least we know it looks good and I can find a little peace in that.

February 23
Day +38

William continues to improve. His blood numbers came

back very good today. His hemoglobin level is 12.5. I don't think it has been over 10.4 since he was diagnosed back in June. He hasn't had blood products in about a week and his numbers continue to rise. This indicates his body is creating blood again. Now we just need to be sure the blood is from the donor's marrow. It will be a few more weeks before we know how well he is grafting. He is still on target to be discharged next week, though he is still on some IV meds right now. The changeover from IV to pill is gradual, but he is doing well with it.

He has been in the hospital for 45 days now, I think he is just tired of being there and is ready to get out!

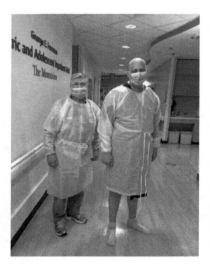

February 24
Day +39

An evening stroll with Grandpa. Did you notice NO IV POLE! I spoke with William's doctor today, and the target discharge day is Wednesday. They are still working with insurance for prescription coverage (there is one medication they don't want to cover). It's a critical medication so that has to be worked out before he can be discharged.

Here is another exciting update. We held several bone marrow drives for William last summer. Three people from those drives have been contacted as matches for patients in need. One person has completed all the steps and is scheduled to harvest stem cells next month. That's what it's all about! Reaching out and helping others. Our job isn't complete; there are more people still looking for their match. When William gets to come home we are planning another drive for blood and bone marrow. Details will be posted at a later date. But heads up: I am hoping to also include a hair drive so start growing out those gorgeous locks! You only need a 6 inch ponytail to donate your hair for a wig for cancer patients!

> *Comment 7: That is awesome. He is doing so good. Amy I had problems with meds from our insurance. We had to get a letter from the doctor for them to cover it. Katie was on an antifungal drug that cost over four thousand dollars. So glad everything is going so good for all of you. God Bless*

> *Comment 9: We had that fight too a couple months back with Voriconizole (or something like that, but it was nearly $4000 a month). But the one they don't want to cover helps prevent GVHD! It's the tacro, and obviously it's critical he gets it!*

> *Comment 43: As other have already mentioned, Lock of Love charges people for the wigs they make, they are not free. So with that in mind, please consider sending your hair donations to a non-profit group called Beautiful Lengths. They are affiliated with the <u>American Cancer Society</u> and people can get FREE wigs through them. <u>http://www.pantene.com/.../beautiful-lengths-about-the...</u> tells more about it. Still praying for William*

February 25
Day +40

OH MY GOD!   THE BOY IS CANCER FREE!
The test results are back...NO LEUKEMIA!

I can barely speak, I can barely type! I am just so thankful
to God for His promises and for His faithfulness!

"Behold I am Jehovah, the God of all flesh. Is there
anything too wonderful for Me?" Jeremiah 32:27

Comment 20: Crying tears of joy for William!!!

*Comment 38: My heart might burst out of my
chest! What wonderful news!!! Praise our God in
heaven above for he is GOOD!*

*Comment 47:   Tried to push "like" more than
once!!!!! Thank u God!!*

*Comment 53: LIKE LIKE LIKE LIKE LIKE!!!! That
is so awesome! I am so, so very happy for you and
for William and for the rest of your family. God is
so good!*

*Comment 75: I'm so happy for u all...your son is
an inspiration to all with his courage and strength*

*Comment 92:   PRAISE THE LORD!!! Don't you
just want to scream it from the rooftops?!! Like I
said before, I don't really know you, and we never
really met, face to face...but we will one day, and
girl you better get ready for a hug!*

*Comment 137: Our God is so incredibly awesome
and amazing! Thank you for sharing your lives*

and your journey with us! As I train this weekend, I will be training in William's honor - with every step raising awareness and funds for blood cancer and blood cancer research! I am so happy your son is cancer free! Praise God!!!!!

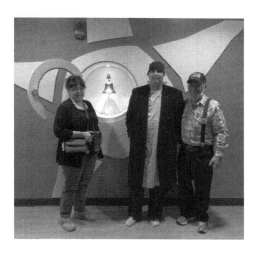

February 26
Day +41

William was discharged today! He had the privilege of ringing the bell. The bell signifies the end of chemo and the beginning of a new life, cancer free! Well done son, well done!

"Ring this bell
Three times well
Its toll to clearly say
My treatment's done
This course I've run
And I am on my way!"

Rear Admiral Irve Charles LeMoyne

Note: If you would like to view the video of the bell binging, it can be seen on William's facebook page, www.facebook.com/hopeforwilliam.

Comment 20: William as you ring the bell I am sure there are many more than me that are wiping tears of love and happiness as our hearts swell because we are SO very proud of you....it is an honor to know such an amazing man that has fought for his own life with such strong faith...God has an amazing plan for you son..I feel it

Comment 22:   I absolutely LOVE seeing him ring that bell! He more than earned it! What a strong, brave young man! You are am inspiration, watching you go through all that you did, but never giving up. You are much stronger than me. William, my hero! God bless you!

Comment 30:   Oh ok now I'm bawling my eyes out...yaaay. praise the Lord

Comment 41:   So excited that he got to ring the bell! This is the best news I have heard all month, and it really made my day. William we are all so proud of you. Your tenacity and spirit definitely paid off!!!

Comment 68:   And I'm crying again, but this time at least it's tears of joy!

Comment 133:   Wonderful! Wonderful! Thank you Lord for hearing our prayers!

What an incredible moment! Watching William ring that bell, it was the miracle we had all prayed and hoped for. As he rang the bell, my heart was full of joy, but also of sadness for the ones who never had this chance. As the bell rang, I thought of Gary, Jenna, Aidan, Zach and the many others who fought so hard but ultimately lost their lives. They had all beat cancer, but died from complications from the transplant. It was a reminder that William wasn't "out of the woods" yet and he still had a long, hard road to recovery ahead of him.

February 27
Day +42

Today William started the daily outpatient portion of his treatment. He goes in every day, including weekends to have his blood, medication and fluid levels checked. He is really happy to be out of the hospital room, and has been enjoying the sunshine between doctor visits.

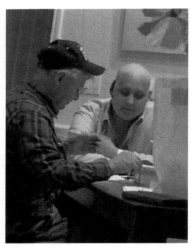

February 28
Day +43

William goes to outpatient appointments every day to have his blood checked and get topped off with any fluids or blood products he might need. Here he is with Grandpa, about to work on a dressing change for his subclavian chest catheter then it will be time to get a little bite to eat, after some meds of course!

March 2
Day +45

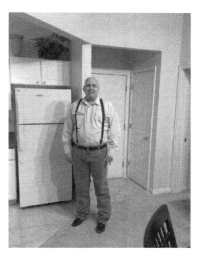

William is doing so well! He spends his mornings in the hospital getting topped off with magnesium and other fluids and getting his blood and medication levels checked. He can do short trips to the store as long as he wears a mask and gloves. He is loving being out of the hospital. Right now he is enjoying soaking up a little sunshine each day and helping me cook. Somehow he also grew an inch or better during his hospital stay. We had to go buy him some jeans today because his old ones were two inches too short.

March 4
Day +47

Today has been a very busy day. Clinic appointment this morning and then we moved into a different apartment this afternoon. Dr. Champlin (stem cell doctor) came by and said his labs are looking excellent! So much so, they are going to drop his clinic appointments down from seven days a week to two. He still has to get IV magnesium, but they said they would arrange a home health company to do that, or I can be trained to do it. I noticed his hair is starting to grow back, and the little stubble he has is white. I mean *white*. I will be curious to see if it stays white or darkens.

We were getting some groceries after we finished moving and I mentioned today was Fat Tuesday. I asked him what he was giving up for Lent. His response, "I'm giving up cancer!"

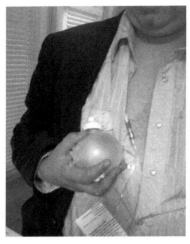

March 5
Day +48

I gave William his magnesium IV today. It feels very strange to be in the home environment and hooking up an IV to a tube hanging out of his chest. Then after the IV, I have to flush the line with saline and heparin. I am still nervous about making sure everything is sterilized right and there are no air bubbles in the syringe. It is a weird feeling knowing everything I put into that line goes straight into his heart...Gee, no pressure there! He usually jokes me through it to lighten the mood.

William is up walking as much as possible. He wants to regain his strength as quickly as possible. Dr. Champlin gave him the go-ahead to start doing some stairs. William said he feels better than he ever has. He has a long recovery still ahead, but he is doing great!

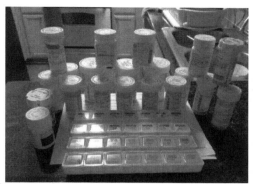

March 9
Day +50

Today is another milestone day. William is at the halfway point of being able to go home. After transplant you have to live within twenty minutes of the hospital for 100 days. Woohoo, halfway there!

Today I had to demonstrate my ability to change the dressing on his catheter, change the caps and flush the lines to a nurse. Now I am officially approved to care for his CVC line at home. Yay!

We got a call this evening that he has tested positive for an active CMV virus so he starts another antiviral, Valcyte to treat it early before it gets out of control. If it does, CMV can attack his internal organs and his eyes, and we don't want it to get there. They will watch him very closely too. Prayers would be appreciated that the meds work fast and attack it quickly since he has no immune system of his own. So with the new medicine added, this is what $42,000 worth of medicines look like! And that's only for one month.

March 11
Day +54

William is still improving. He talked to Dr. Champlin

today about the possibility of getting off steroids and maybe going home a little earlier than the usual 100 days. He is doing well enough that the doctor started weaning him off the steroids today (YAY!). He will evaluate William at day +90 and if he is still doing well, the doctor will consider letting him return home sooner. To be honest we are all getting impatient, and are ready to get back home. Even day +90 is still ten days sooner. We'll take it if he allows it.

March 14
Day +57

I have teased William that I think an alien has abducted the real William. This morning he woke up at 5:45 a.m., took his meds, made me breakfast in bed (and didn't burn my omelet), did the dishes and then ironed his shirt.

It is like a miracle has taken place! All kidding aside, it wasn't that long ago that we weren't even sure if William was going to make it, and look at him now.

March 16
Day +59

William told me yesterday that his biggest fear is to reach up and touch his neck and feel the "chain" again. The chain is the swollen lymph nodes in the neck, and if it returns, it could signify his cancer has returned. I told him that it's a normal fear and it would stay with him for a long time. But that got me thinking about how cancer has changed us. There is a veil of security that has been ripped from us. It may have been a false security to begin with, but be honest with yourself, how many of you have really thought cancer would affect YOUR child? Before this happened I never really thought it would happen to us, and now there is a fear that is always in the back of my mind. I fear William relapsing. I fear one of my other children being diagnosed. Maybe in time these fears will subside but I truly doubt they will ever go away.

At the same time, this fear almost forces you to step back and see what matters most. If you knew ahead of time you only had a small amount of time left with your family, what would you do? How would you spend that time? The answer isn't the same for everyone, but for William and me, it was to talk. Just to spend time together and talk. Some nights we talked so late! A lot of what we talked about I never posted. Some of the things are just too painful to verbalize. We talked about his relationship with God and his eternal security. We talked about what he wanted to do with his body if he died, and we planned his funeral. The worst part was knowing there was a good chance I would have to see his wishes through. It was just by the grace of God I didn't!

William shared something with me the other day. He told me one night when he was in the hospital, during the worst; he felt death was near him. He could feel it and wasn't strong enough to fight it. He then felt a hand gently touch him on his forehead and peace overtook him. He opened his eyes, and no one was there but he said he could physically feel the hand of God on him, though he couldn't see Him. After he told me that, I then told him how I had prayed for him. As he progressively got worse, I just prayed for God to reach down and touch him and heal him. Some people say God doesn't do miracles anymore but I beg to differ. This whole journey has been full of miracles, and the hand of God has been with us the entire time.

"And the peace of God, which surpasses all understanding, will guard your hearts and your minds in Christ Jesus." (Philippians 4:7 ESV)

Comment 5: I'm amazed at the strength you have had through this journey with your son . I can't imagine what it's like .. But my mother's diagnosis has brought us closer and we've had " that" talk. I hope I haven't left anything unsaid, and I know that she knows how much I love her... And when her journey is OVER, I'm ok with it, because tomorrow , it will be my turn. Thank you, for allowing us this journey, through a "Mother's eyes". Prayers continued for you and family!! I read your entries , through William's journey to my mother .... It brought a HUGE smile to her face!!! She said" through God, all things are possible"!!!! Amen to that.

Comment 9: Yes the same thing happened to me 25 years ago...and William will look at life totally different. He will walk up to a stranger and know that he too is going thru a difficult time and he will just give him a hug. God has given us a gift....life

Comment 27: As a mother of a daughter who has had cancer, I can say that whatever you are feeling, were the same feelings I had. unfortunately, my relationship with god has come to an end, cancer in my family has changed me forever. BUT, I read about William with interest, hope and love, that YOU William will get better and go from strength to strength. keep smiling my lovely. Xx

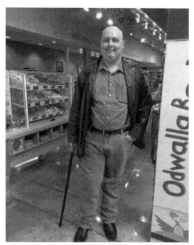

March 18
Day +61

William had an outing to the local Whole Foods to pick up some organic, GMO free food. Even though we will never know why he ended up with leukemia, William and I both think environmental issues contributed to it (such as chemicals and unnatural things in food). With that, he wants to eat less processed foods and more organic and non GMO foods. He said he would do whatever it takes to keep from going through that again!

He continues to get better; today his doctor took him off the steroids that he hates so much! And he was able to drop a second medication too. Two down, twenty more to go. Hey, it's a start!

> *Comment 4: You look great William!! I think you are smart with your food choices. As a 6 year survivor, I too am careful with my food including going gluten free. Another good idea is to be sure you're using non toxic cleaning products in your home. The less chemicals breathed in, the better*

> *Comment 10: And he is not having to wear a mask outside!!!!*

> *Comment 18: Love the idea of going organic and gmo free! We did the same thing when our son was*

diagnosed with a brain tumour! We are still doing it, it's an adjustment, but well worth it!!

Comment 49: Mask up <u>Hope for William</u>! You have a suppressed immune system. Any illness can put you back in the hospital! I wear mine all the time! Looking great! Stay strong and positive! The Ladybug Warrior.

March 19
Day +62

I have a quick prayer request, William's CMV (virus) is proving to be stubborn. The antivirals are not really giving us the results his doctor was looking for. It hasn't gotten any worse, but it hasn't gotten any better. They took him off Valcyte today and moved him to an IV antiviral, Gancyclovir, twice a day. So now he gets three IV's a day (one magnesium and two doses of the antiviral). He is not symptomatic or acting sick at all, which is good but we still need the virus gone.

March 21
Day +64

Grrrr! William's CMV just isn't playing by the rules! It hasn't improved yet. Hopefully a few more days on the IV antivirals and by Tuesday's clinic appointment we will see some improvement. He ended up needing platelets today, the first time in about five weeks he has needed blood products. His nurse said his numbers dropped from both the CMV and the medicines for it. I really hope this infection gets under control quickly, it's beginning to concern me. I also know how bad William wants to go home and this will throw a serious wrench in his plans.

March 24
Day +67

William took his Survivorship Class today. It was a guide to living with the new restrictions of his life. He learned the schedule for getting his childhood vaccines all over, food restrictions - even vitamin restrictions, the information that needs to be on his medic alert bracelet, specific type of sunglasses to help protect him from eye cancer and pages upon pages of information! I will get to look through it when I get back this weekend, but he called after the class to tell me some of the highlights. My parents are with him now so they were able to take the class with him too. It was a lot of information.

Tomorrow he goes for labs and a clinic appointment. I really hope and pray the CMV virus is responding to the IV meds and the active infection is going away. The IV comes with its own set of side effects that are causing problems for him. Overall he is still doing well, just a few little hurdles he still needs to get over.

From William's journal:

"Now I've been out patient for over a month now, and even though I have CMV, VRE and GVHD and take roughly 30-35 pills a day and take three at-home IV's, I am feeling great! I'm out walking around and going places and enjoying every minute of it! Today is 67 days post transplant, and I am walking again with no cane, no walker and no wheelchair. It's blown me away how fast you can recover from something as hard and debilitating as the transplant is and was. The only way I can describe it is, it's like a baptism of fire. You can feel the chemo pulsing through your veins. It feels like your whole body, both inside and out is engulfed in flames. Even though I couldn't see it at the time there was and always will be a silver lining!"

March 26
Day +68

This has been a very emotional week for me. I was able to come back home while my parents stayed with William. I have tried to catch up on phone calls, get a house ready to sell, do taxes, get my hair cut, pay bills and get ready to go back to Houston this weekend. I will be bringing James and Abbey with me. I have shown them all the pictures of William, and how sick he looked, and that he is bald again to help prepare them. The last time they saw William his hair was growing back, and Abbey is still too young to understand what is happening. It scares her when he is bald. Both James and Abbey have reached the point that every time I have to leave them for a week or two, they go into the "Missing Mommy Meltdowns" so I decided to bring them with me. I have no idea how I am going to do this. They can't go into certain areas of the hospital because they are too young.

Even though I have stayed busy, it seems I have lost the ability to outrun my emotions! While Tara was working on my hair yesterday, she, my sister, and I were talking about William and I actually voiced his final wishes for the first time. I was not able to choke the actual words out of my mouth until yesterday. Maybe I just couldn't stand the thought of hearing them spoken because it made it more real, but for whatever reason I have held his wishes in my heart since August because I couldn't speak them out loud.

So much of what William has gone through, I have shared openly. I did this for a reason. When William was first diagnosed I didn't know what to expect and no one was really able to prepare us for what was coming. You kind of know chemo causes nausea and your hair falls out but beyond that - nothing! I have been pretty open with his physical trials and triumphs, and I have been open about my fears, anger, faith and hope. It is *all* a part of the journey and I wanted anyone reading this to know what the real face of cancer looks like because sometimes I thought what I was feeling was wrong until I heard another person say they felt the same way. Even though some days my faith was really strong, there were days I wanted to look up in the sky and scream F*** YOU CANCER! And guess what? There were a few days I actually did.

Yesterday William went to his Survivorship Class. Mom called me this morning and gave me some more details about it. William has sustained damage to all of his organs from the months of chemo. His life won't ever go back to the "old normal." He will have a lot of restrictions now. Some will only last 6 months, some will last for a few years and some will be life-long. One thing he was told is that he will always have to wear sunglasses (even on cloudy days) to protect himself from eye cancer. Remember when his skin turned black and peeled off? The protective coating on his eyes did too. He will have to wash his clothes in a Sun Guard to make his clothes have SPF 50 to help protect his skin from skin cancer. His lungs sustained enough damage that he will be susceptible to pneumonia for the rest of his life. There are just pages and pages of things we need to do and learn. While it is all so overwhelming, I am also so grateful to MD Anderson. His Survivorship nurse said a lot of this information is new and based on his test results specifically. It will be different for each person, but his guidelines are tailored to him alone. That's a pretty intense level of care!

William saw his doctor today too, and his CMV level dropped to 3. This is awesome news! They are keeping him on the IV anti-viral for a little bit longer because it is working. This is great news! I have more to say but it's getting late and I have two little ones that need to go to bed. So that's all for tonight.

> *Comment 7: Thank you for I am a survivor of cancer I fought for 2 long yrs and I myself have some long lasting things too like my heart it is not that of 27 yr old it's more like 60 yr old I am not able to do some things as well as eat some things I taste metal all the time like I am eating a penny but I wear my badge of honor bc there were so many that didn't make it!!! I pray that you feel some since of peace with him*

> *Comment 43: Beautiful emotions, and all the more poignant because you have shared them so openly with all of us who are a part of this journey with you. You and William are amazing human beings, and somehow, somewhere, there will be some good that comes from this. William will give hope to so many others, and that is a very precious thing.*

> *Comment 45: I know all of this sounds hard, but it will become habit. And you eventually just do it without thinking. My body has went threw a lot, I wore my mask at home..oh my that was a hassle but I had to do it. I have 4 kids that go to 3*

different schools..lots of germs. And still I've gotten sick..ugh!!! When you need to scream F cancer! Do it, we all feel that way sometimes! Chemo is such a harsh drug, my kidneys will never be the same. But I'll take it over the cancer. You got this! Prayers continue!

Comment 53: U know i have been where u are....at least for a short time anyway. U write so well. Thank u for being so honest & sharing ur journey. I've needed to read this & re-feel incomplete emotions

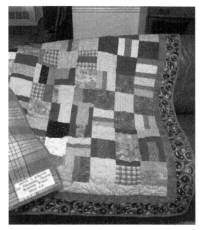

March 27
Day +69

This beautiful, double sided quilt came in the mail yesterday from Stitches and Prayers at First Christian Church in Rowlett. It is beautiful and I don't even know who to thank! If you are on this site please know, the quilt is absolutely gorgeous and we truly appreciate it. Quilting is such a beautiful art. I will be heading back to Houston this weekend and will take the quilt to William. I did send him a picture of it and he said "WOW!" I told him the picture doesn't do it justice, wait till he sees it!

As I had mentioned the other day, this week has been an emotional one! Two people died of leukemia this week. One adult, and one child. Another child was newly diagnosed. I am members of several leukemia groups on

Facebook. Since William was diagnosed at least one person dies a week. Some weeks as many as three die. It is awful! To open your newsfeed and hope and pray you are going to get a good update only to find the person you have held in your heart has "earned their angel wings" is crushing. I don't know what hurts the worst though, reading about another warrior getting their angel wings or reading a new diagnosis post. I cry at every one. I cry because I know the crushing pain and paralyzing fear that parent has! I cry because the odds SUCK for their child! I cry because I know what's coming for their child and there is *no nice way* to warn them! And in the groups, we do warn them. We have to be up front and honest because there is no reason to sugar-coat it. These moms and dads are warriors too. They have helped me so much. They have lifted me out of some deep pits and given me hope, even in some of the darkest moments.

I saw a post the other day, it was a video. A little girl was getting a new Barbie, named Ella. Ella is a chemo Barbie. She is bald and comes with two wigs and a head scarf. The little girl was about four or five with long blonde hair and she was about to start chemo. Her mom was explaining that Ella's hair fell out because of the chemo. And the little girl asked if her hair was going to fall out all at once or a little at a time. I just bawled. The post was a petition to Mattel to create more Ella Barbies because there aren't enough of them for all the little kids going through chemo. It wasn't a commercial, it was an actual video of an actual little girl with leukemia, and it devastated me. Probably because this is real, so many people, so many kids and I just wish it would stop! The reality is though, that leukemia diagnosis are supposed to increase 43% in the next year!

I think one of the reasons this was such an emotional week was because I was back home and things were "normal" for a while, and I think the emotions of the last nine months have started catching up with me. I think hearing about William's organ damage was part of it too. In your mind, you think "once we get to transplant, it will be okay." You forget the chemo (and months upon months of it) slowly leaves a permanent mark on the body. And don't get me wrong, I am forever grateful for every extra day I get with William, but I also know he has sustained permanent damage that will affect him the rest of his life. And while I am grateful, I am mad too! William is a good kid and he didn't deserve this!

I keep thinking about the apostle Paul, he pleaded with the Lord three times to remove the thorn in his flesh and the Lord said to him "My grace is sufficient for you, my strength is made perfect in weakness." We don't know what Paul's thorn was, and it doesn't matter. He had "issues" and we all do, but even with our issues, if we are willing, God can still use us in big ways.

I don't know why this happened to William, and probably never will know. For whatever reason, William was allowed to bear this. And somehow God will see him through it with His grace and strength.

> *Comment 4: Beautiful Amy. It is hard to look on those sites and like you said either someone has earned their wings or they are being told they have this dreaded disease. I said they same thing about Katie she was always a good girl never gave me any trouble. I felt guilty for a long time because I brought her in this world and I use to say if I hadn't had her she wouldn't be going through this. But it has made us both stronger and my faith is a*

lot stronger. Chemo left Katie with heart damage and kidney problems but they are getting better. The doctors told Katie she could have children but she said momma if I want kids I can adopt because they're a lot of kids that needs a home. I thank God she is still with me. But I don't know if I will ever get to where I use to be before she got sick. I know I don't take anything for granted anymore. Tell William hello for us and we are so thankful he is doing so good. God Bless

Comment 7: I cried while reading the entire letter. I cry every time I see someone with cancer. Since it has touched my family I will never be the same. My faith was challenged. My mourning increased. But I still believe in a miracle working God and He can heal any damaged organ that chemo has touched. I still proclaim and decree William restored totally to complete resurrected health. Every organ , eyes, any damage line up with the word of God and he be healed by the stripes of Jesus. I expect nothing less. I pray for supernatural strength in you precious Amy. I lost a brother, but this is your son whom you carried in your womb. I can't compare the hurt. My heart hurts but rejoices with you. This too shall pass.

Comment 8: Amen to that. As you probably know by now, I am 10 years out. Yes, my eyes still bother me, I do get skin cancers (basil cell) and see the Dermatologist every 6 months, I continually have heartburn and cannot eat after 6 pm, or I can't sleep because of the heartburn, I am out of breath more often than not...etc.. but seriously, I consider this all MINOR side effects. I play golf, snow ski, dance and drink wine..William has a full and glorious life ahead of him. Like me, he is one of the lucky ones..praise to you, lord Jesus Christ

Comment 19: How very difficult it is. I know my sweet daughter went to heaven 11 years ago it was cancer that took her from me. I am so thankful William is still here for you to hold and Love ! Blessings

Comment 29: God bless you. I just continually ask the question, "WHY is this happening and just increasing?" There has to be a reason. I don't understand.

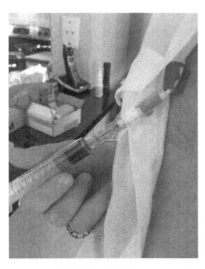

March 29
Day +72

William has taken charge of his medications and administers his own IV's too. He was showing me that his nurse told him he needs to check the blood return before each IV (he does three a day), to make sure the line is flowing right. So he pulls the blood into the syringe and shows me. I told him "Okay I see it, now put it back!"

Yesterday his platelets were really low and he had to get a transfusion. He has to go back an extra day next week to get checked again. It's the IV antiviral causing his numbers to drop. Hopefully he can get off of them soon because its affecting his white cell count too, and if that drops too low he will need Neupogen shots in his stomach again. They hurt and he hates them!

March 30
Day+73

William is finally playing guitar again. When he lost his skin, he lost his calluses too. His new skin is very tender and he can only play for short periods. He has to be careful not to play till his fingers bleed, like he did when he first learned to play. He said now he has a "player's mind with beginner fingers." James and Abbey are enjoying him playing again, and don't seem to be quite as nervous around him.

Tomorrow he gets his platelets checked and we meet with the nutritionist so we can learn how he will have to change his diet to help his damaged organs. His heart and lungs are only at 50%, over time he will be able to increase to about 70%, but it will be a few years. His kidneys and liver are also damaged but not to the degree of his heart and lungs. It's just collateral damage from months of chemo. He accepts it pretty well, and hopes to achieve the full 70% or more but understands some things will never be the same, and that's ok.

April 1
Day +75

William's platelets have just arrived, and it's a single donor bag. Yay! Those are so much better for the patient than a "mixed bag." A mixed bag is where they pull platelets out of a whole blood donation and combine the platelets from three or four different donors.

The best news is he has had two negative CMV readings in a row. One more and he can get off the IV med. Then his blood numbers should rebound and hold steady again, as they were before he got the CMV virus. His other labs are looking good and his doctor is very pleased with his progress.

Today as we were waiting for William's blood draw, I saw so many people in wheelchairs being taken from one appointment to the next. This was William just a few short months ago, and now he is up walking without his walker or even his cane. It's amazing how far he has come in 10 months!

April 2
Day +76

William's doctor finally allowed him to introduce frozen fruits and cooked vegetables back into his diet. Every day since then he has enjoyed yogurt and fruit smoothies.

William and I both want to give a shout-out to a friend of his. We have another hero in our midst! Phillip is one of William's childhood friends and he joined the bone marrow registry in hopes of being a match for William. He received notice he is a match for another person and he is going to donate. Speaking from experience on the recipient side, you are giving a family the greatest possible gift. You are giving hope and you are giving life!

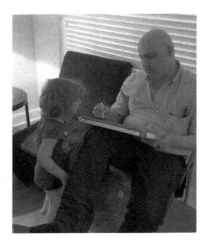

April 4
Day +78

William had a very long day at MDA today. He got more platelets today and did his full panel of lung tests so we know the extent of the chemo damage to his lungs. The damage there is permanent and will not heal itself over time. It's livable but means he will always have to take precautions and be very careful to guard against pneumonia, which he will be prone to for the rest of his life. He has the lungs of a 70 year old, to put it in perspective.

Back at the apartment, his little brother and sister have sweet-talked him into watching *My Little Pony* with them and they are drawing pictures of dinosaurs and bats for each other on the MagnaDoodle. As I sit back and look on the scene, all is right in my world! He made it, he survived! And I am enjoying having all of my kids under one roof, even if it is just for a short while.

April 5
Day +79

William is not having a good day! He slipped and fell last night and hurt his knee and the toenail that he is going to lose started bleeding. Today he has had to stay in bed with his feet and legs elevated and iced. His platelets and white blood cells are low (from the CMV medicine), and he is having some rectal bleeding issues as well. One of the terrible side effects of chemo that you don't hear about too often is what it does to hemorrhoids. William has been having problems with hemorrhoids since his first dose of chemo back in June. They have progressively gotten worse. Even the prescription medications don't offer much relief. Every time his white cells and platelets drop, they bleed. We have to be careful of how much he bleeds when the platelets drop. Right now he has it under control but if he starts bleeding heavier we will have to go to the ER. He is also nauseated again too, he took his first nausea pill in almost three months! ☹

April 7
Day +81

William has been sleeping a lot the last few days but he says he feels okay. I think it is from the medicines, especially the IV medicine. I will be glad when he gets off that one, he will be too. His toenail is looking better. Tomorrow is a clinic appointment, hoping for a good visit.

April 10
Day +84

We have had a very busy week! William had a long clinic visit earlier in the week. Almost all his labs are "off" and they really aren't sure why. They finally took him off the IV since he has had four negative CMV tests (yay!), so his blood numbers should rebound and stay steady.

He is nearing the magic 100 day mark, where he can return home. As I mentioned in an earlier post, we were getting a house ready to sell. We got an offer on the house before we even had a chance to list it. We closed on the house this week and William's doctor allowed me to bring him home for a short trip (with very strict guidelines). I think the trip home did wonders for him! He has been in almost total isolation since December; he really needed this! I would ask for prayers for traveling mercies though. My dad is taking him back to Houston right now, so please pray for a safe trip back. I will return early next week, so keep me in your prayers too please.

April 11
Day +85

Another day, another bag of platelets! Except for the blood numbers, William's other labs leveled out. The blood will rebuild slowly now that he is off the IV meds for the CMV. His white cell count is low so he had to get more shots in the stomach to help boost those.

Some of the emotional aspects of what he has been through are beginning to hit him pretty hard right now. There is something called survivor guilt that he is experiencing. Losing his friend, Gary (back in December) has made it more real. They were supposed to get through this together and encourage each other along the way. We even planned to have a big BBQ when they were both back home to celebrate their recoveries. But even though Gary's family will be with us at that BBQ, Gary won't. William feels grateful he survived, but also guilty. It's very common, but a heavy load for someone his age to deal with. All of this has been a heavy load!

> Comment 8: Love and strength to you Amy and to William. I hope he can let the guilt go and that he knows his survival gives him the opportunity to

help others in this life. He is important to so many, Mack and I included. Xxx

Comment 13: William, don't be sad. God brings his children home in His time. I lost my son, Colin. 4 years ago, and through prayer have come to understand that He created this world for us, but our days are numbered in His book. But you will live to fight another day. He wants you to be here. Feel blessed, my friend. I guarantee you that the love that surrounds your friends and my son in Heaven is greater than anything here. They are singing and dancing in Heaven. Fight on.

Comment 21: It is tough. We all experience this and 10 years later, I still ask why me? Why did I survive. Live life to the fullest. Never forget your buds. They all are your guardian Angels now.

April 12
Day +86

Today has been a busy, but relaxing. William's nutrition team said he needs to be on a "plant based" diet with minimal meats. William decided that instead of being a naughty vegetarian, he was going all in. But he is still limited on what fruits and veggies he can eat, and they have to be prepared a special way. I spent today making and freezing vegetarian lasagna, frittata and zucchini muffins. His little brother is allergic to dairy so I made up some dairy free meals for him too. Dad is with William right now and the kids and I head back Tuesday to stay with William until he gets to return home for good. So I have been cooking and sending pictures to William of what

I am bringing him. He can't do too much right now because his feet and legs are so swollen they look deformed. Hopefully by Tuesday the swelling will go down. The skin hurts from being stretched!

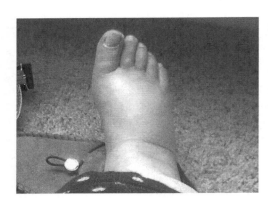

April 13
Day +87

All right y'all, the swelling is getting worse in William's feet and ankles. He is really hurting and walking is incredibly painful. He needs some serious prayers for the swelling to subside...and quickly!

Comment 6: The doctors gave me a prescription for a diuretic before I left the hospital to prevent the swelling. He needs to call the doctor because it can cause him to go into congestive heart failure.

Comment 7: I know all cases are different but watch for a dry cough and shortness of breath

Comment 23: Get him some good compression socks too! That will work out some of the swelling. Poor William. Praying and sending positive thoughts your way. Xo

Comment 31: Please get him on a diuretic - it will relieve it very quickly. Elevating the feet will only help a little and could make the fluid load on his other organs worse. This is easily resolved with a diuretic - and borrow a urine bottle for him to use at first until his feet are less swollen (until they are not painful). Xxxxx

Comment 49: LASIK is wonderful and keep those legs ELEVATED higher than his heart.

April 15
Day +89

William's feet are much better! They are not completely back to normal but they are getting there. His doctor didn't want to put him on Lasik because he is on a beta blocker to slow his heart rate. Adding any kind of water pill could slow his heart too much. He is back on L-glutamine, and that helps the swelling a lot!

The kids and I made it safely back to Houston, and Dad is on his way back home. For now, it looks like April 26 is the target date for William to return home. A bone marrow biopsy has been scheduled for this Friday, so please pray for no leukemia cells. The target date could change depending on results from this biopsy, but more important than going home is for him to still be cancer-free!

April 17
Day +91

Tomorrow William has his bone marrow biopsy and some heart tests. I will be nervous until we get the results. We have about a week left before William finally gets to return home. He is beyond ready! The little ones are too; it's been a rough trip for Abbey. She fell and hit her mouth on the coffee table, we were very lucky she didn't knock a few teeth out.

Even though we are all ready to go home, there is a level of comfort being here that I am going to miss. If anything happens, William is literally 1.6 miles from MDA. Last week, when his doctor allowed him to make the quick trip back home I was a nervous wreck. What if he spikes a fever? What if his counts drop? What if he falls? What if, what if, what if?

I don't know if he is going to have his chest catheter removed or if he goes home with it. Obviously I have some questions and maybe a tad bit of anxiety too.

> *Comment 3: Don't think that way....turn it around...you are worrying about healing he has already been given...the devil is making you doubt God's ability to keep that promise....look how far he has come...be thankful....and not worried...let God do his work....still praying and still believing !!!*

> *Comment 4: Prayers.....just remember to breathe and enjoy every single second. You can't live in fear...you might miss something wonderful!! Keep up the good work, William!!!*

April 18
Day +92

Today has not been so great. Actually, it has just been a bad day. William is still at the hospital, now going on twelve hours. All his blood numbers took a dive today, and he is getting red blood and platelets again today. His doctor is puzzled at what caused the drastic drop, especially this late in the game. This could stop him from coming home next week too. Just hearing that news completely crushed his spirits.

We see his transplant doctor on Monday, and will go over today's labs and hopefully have the preliminary bone marrow results by then. They will run more labs and add extra appointments for next week to monitor the labs and determine if he can come home or not.

It is emotionally devastating to be this close to the end and hit a road block like this! There is the obvious worry of *why* his numbers did this, and there is the complete and total exhaustion of being away from home for so long. Even my little ones are having a rough time. We are all exhausted physically, emotionally and mentally.

> *Comment 2: Things looked really dark on a Friday 2,000 or so years ago....but everything changed by Sunday! Praying!*

> *Comment 7: So many prayers....i am so sorry about his counts, i know how scary it is!! There are reasons this happens, and i hope they figure it out...its so hard not having answers. Please know i think about you and william so much and he is in my prayers. I know he is probably so angry right now, so close to going home. It seems that's when these things happen...when looking forward to something. Hang in there - lots of love and prayers!*

> *Comment 10: William IS proof of God's tremendous love and benevolence and we pray every day believing God will continue to use him*

as a testimony of His awesome power and healing! Keep the faith through these dark days-so many prayers and love for you and your family who have been through so much!

Comment 39: There will be bumps along the road. He is allowed some crush time but only a short time. He will come through. He mental attitude now is as key as the physical recovery. Prayers from Cincy.

Comment 45: Don't get discouraged God can do all things!! When you're at your lowest He is right on time!!!

Comment 46: Jesus died on this Easter weekend AND rose from the dead so that we can have life like His...whole, complete, and healed! Claim your healing now and call it forth despite what you see. God will hear and answer and manifest complete healing in His time as you continue to speak out your healing and rest in Him. Resting in Him is your strongest weapon against the opposition coming again you for greater is He within than the enemy in the world! You all with Papa God have got this!!

Comment 53: This happens often. Please don't despair. I went home, only to have to go back less than a week later. There are going to be many many difficult moments, many disappointments and challenges. Very few get to go home after 100 days. Stay there until it is completely safe and embrace the journey, or you will have a very difficult time of it. I completely understand the frustration, I've been there, but looking back, it was all worth it. Blessings to you and yours. Happy Easter.

Comment 55: I promise them road bumps will come & go! I just had to restart on some of my immune suppressing drugs, because I took infection. So I have to be on all of them again. And soooo close to a year! But just another bump in the road! Prayers continue!

Comment 56: to William and his family, keep your spirit's up. its a long road that you all walk together with it's twists and turns, it will be an emotional, physical and mentally difficult and no two days will be the same. sending you all hugs and best wishes. xx

April 21
Day +95

William is getting two units of blood today. His hemoglobin levels were still pretty low. His doctor wants to see him again on Thursday to check his labs again. Dr. Champlin wants to speak personally to William's at-home doctor to discuss routine lab checks. If he can do that by Thursday and if William's labs are ok, he will release him to go home. We will still come back to MDA every three months for scheduled tests, but his weekly lab works and transfusions will be done local. Dr. Champlin doesn't seem overly concerned about the recent drop in blood numbers; he believes it is from the IV med for his CMV infection. He said it takes a solid two weeks to get out of the system.

His preliminary bone marrow reports show 1% blasts. My heart fell when I heard it until I remembered that anything under 2% is good. The doctor was happy about the preliminary results and said he will call with the final results, but expects it to be good news.

God is good! He took a sick and dying young man, with no hope of living and through the blood of another, gave him new life.

> *Comment 1: Actually, He gave him a Mom willing to fight without end until the powers of this earth submitted to her power...which you are a vessel for Him!*

> *Comment 3: Greater is He that is in you then he that is in the World. All the Glory goes to Jesus our healer and intercessor . So excited. Closer to my dance with William. Give him huge kiss from me and hug from Jim*

> *Comment 4: Wow! That last statement is not just William's story, but the story of the gospel. God took a sick and dying, sinful humanity, and through the blood of Jesus, gave those who receive Him new life! Still praying for you all and for William to stay encouraged.*

> *Comment 11: I THINK WE NEED A BIG "AMEN" TO THIS POST! AND ALL GOD'S CHILDREN SAID......"AMEN!"*

April 23
Day +97

You know that feeling you get right before a vacation? Your mind has already "checked out" but physically you still have to be there, and time just creeps by. That's where we are now! Day 100 is just around the corner and we are so close to being able to go home.

William sees Dr. Champlin tomorrow morning, and will have his labs checked. His blood numbers have been really low the past several weeks. I really hope his body is rebounding and rebuilding now. We expect to be discharged to return home tomorrow, but what time we leave will depend on if he needs blood or not. We also need to discuss returning home with his chest catheter. Since he is still requiring regular blood and platelets, William kind of wants to keep it in for now. He isn't very keen on IV's and they can draw his blood for his labs out of the catheter too. It keeps him from having arm pricks twice a week. We will see what Dr Champlin says tomorrow.

Upon the return home, William will go to his local oncologist twice a week to check his labs and get blood as needed. Once he no longer requires blood on a routine basis he will drop to once a week until the six month mark. Then we come back to MDA for more tests and they will begin to wean him off some of his immune suppression medicines. But one step at a time...right now we just need to get home. Home sweet home!

April 25
Day +99

Guess where we are? HOME!

We got here late last night. Normally I don't drive at night but we were so anxious to get home, I drank lots of coffee and we hit the road. William had platelets yesterday (his were very low), and ended up being at the hospital for over ten hours. We had the apartment packed and ready to load. So as soon as we left the hospital, we loaded the van and hit the road.

On Monday he sees his local oncologist to have his labs checked and will probably get more platelets. Dr. Champlin decided to leave his catheter in for now since he is requiring blood transfusions twice a week. It's just easier and much less painful to use the catheter than to do an IV at every visit. That plus he is neutropenic so every time his skin is broken, he is susceptible to infection.

We go back to MDA on May 22 for another bone marrow biopsy and maybe to remove the chest catheter at that time. William rested today. He has been tired. He said he feels okay - not bad, but not good either. A few days of rest may be good for him. He has had two very long hospital days this week and a long drive. I am just catching up on errands. It feels good to get caught up. If William feels up to it, I will get a picture of him tomorrow and post it, his hair is starting to grow back a little bit. I didn't want to pester him today for a picture while he is so tired.

April 28
Day 102

Wahoo, good news at the appointment today! Dad took William to his local oncologist for lab checks. All of his blood numbers rose significantly. If his numbers continue upwards he will be able to drop to one appointment a week.

May 1
Day +105

No such luck, William had a rough day at the clinic! His blood numbers dropped again, which meant he needed platelets and red blood. The red blood order didn't get entered in time so he has to go back tomorrow morning for the red blood. They did get the platelets done today. It was just a harsh reminder that the road to recovery is going to be a very long one, full of ups and downs.

William has been struggling emotionally for months now and asked me today if I would set him up to see a counselor. Many people who survive cancer or transplants end up dealing with Survivor's Guilt and/or Post Traumatic Stress Disorder. We keep reminding him that all these feelings are normal. But I agree with him, and I think it is time he sees a professional to help him cope with all the emotions, fear and anxieties he is having. Even though I have walked *with* him through this journey, I have not actually walked *in* his shoes, so I can't truly understand the emotions he is going through.

May 2
Day +106

William received more blood today, so he should be good for the weekend. We went out to the back porch and had a little target practice with his air soft gun (if you see him, ask him who the best shot was!). He just said he wants a rematch tomorrow! Lol

May 7
Day +111

William has been doing okay lately. Not really great, still needing blood, and today he threw up a little. I have noticed him mentioning stomach issues more than once or twice lately so we are staying closely connected with MD Anderson, as well as his local doctor and he is being very closely watched for signs of the GVHD returning. He has another doctor appointment tomorrow.

Right now we are all still settling in and re-adjusting to the newest "norm." Last week I sat down and starting combing through the grocery ads for sale prices on organic fruits and vegetables. I realized that was the first time in eleven months I had been able to do that! I was so happy I couldn't stop smiling. It is amazing how much we take for granted, but in that moment I knew I was blessed beyond measure. My entire family was back under one roof and my biggest concern for the moment was who had the cheapest price on zucchini. For that moment, no thoughts of cancer, or relapse, or death, or funeral plans entered my mind. Just a quiet moment reading the paper, and I will never take those precious peaceful moments for granted again!

> *Comment 6: So happy that you have had your first moment of "normal" and not worrying - hope that William just starts improving every day and that soon your 'normal' is normal and your worries are few! Xxx*

> *Comment 11: Isn't it great when you notice you just did something without even thinking about "it?" sometimes i can do something for like three hours without it taking over my thoughts! It's*

amazing what you have been through and are standing on the other side. William is amazing!! I am so so happy he is doing well!

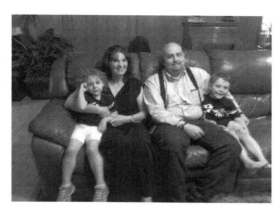

May 11
Day +115

I want to wish all the moms a Happy Mother's Day today. For me, this is a very special day. My sister-in-law said it best; when she hugged William today she said it was like hugging a miracle!

We changed William's treatment hospital this week. One of the major issues with cancer or transplant patients is the fact they have weakened immune systems. When they need to go to the ER, if there is not a separate entrance for them, they sit in a waiting room surrounded by people with infections. These infections can become life threatening. The new hospital will isolate transplant patients upon arrival, to help protect them from being exposed to germs and infections.

May 16
Day +120

William has been a couple weeks without needing blood products. We are going back to MD Anderson next week

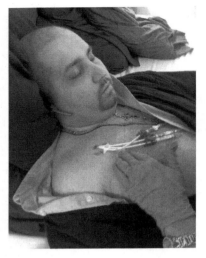

for follow ups, chest x-rays and another bone marrow biopsy. Hopefully his blood numbers will remain steady now. If so, he can have his chest catheter removed next week while we are at MDA. That will be a huge milestone in this journey.

May 22
Day +126

We are back at MD Anderson. Today's appointments went well. William's blood numbers are still holding steady. He can finally drop his lab/blood checks to once a week! Tomorrow he has his bone marrow biopsy very early in the morning, and then we will be heading back home. His doctor wants to keep his chest catheter in until he gets the results from the biopsy, just in case anything comes back unusual. The doctor doesn't expect anything like that, but he said he would rather be double sure. So hopefully it will be removed in a week or so. He said his doctor in Dallas can take it out.

For the first time in almost a year I feel relief! Dr. Champlin said he needs to do his weekly lab check at home but he doesn't need to return to MDA for 2 months. Wow! In the last year we have spent more time in Houston than at home, and two months is *huge*. We can actually unpack our bags! Ah, yes, it is the little things that make you happy!

Have a safe Memorial Day weekend everyone, especially if you are traveling.

May 27
Day +131

Preliminary results from the bone marrow biopsy are showing ZERO % blasts! It will be a week before we have final results but this is awesome! Once final results are in, if everything looks good, William can finally get the CVC (chest catheter) out. His blood has been holding steady and NO CANCER CELLS! Good news, good news, good news!

> *Comment 7: Dance in heaven for me Gary. Kiss my Lord's feet for this miracle of life for your precious friend. I know you've been praying up there.*

> *Comment 10:   "Like" just doesn't cover it! LOVE!!!!!!!!!!!!!!!!!!!!!!!!!!!!!!!!!!!!!*

> *Comment 42: Praise the Lord! What great news! Still Rockin' Orange for William!*

May 31
Day +135

Well, crap! William has tested positive for influenza 3 and is on his way to the emergency room for chest x-rays, evaluation, etc. He has no immune system so this could turn ugly fast. Lots and lots of prayers please!

June 1
Day +136

William does not have pneumonia. The flu is the only infection he has. They ran an extensive panel of tests to make sure there were no secondary infections. He stays on a regimen of antiviral, antibacterial and antifungal medications, and it appears when he caught this flu virus his antibiotics worked exactly as they needed to. Since he has no immune system of his own, these pills are all he has...and they worked. The virus is mild and the doctor called in an additional antibiotic and some cough meds. William did not have to be admitted, but he is on fever watch and pneumonia symptom watch. His doctor also said he needs to stay INSIDE the house while allergies are high as this will increase his chance of pneumonia. So basically William is back in isolation.

Visitors will need to be kept at a minimum and will need to be scheduled through Aunt Kelly again. William's system is weakened so we are not taking any chances. If Kelly approves you to visit please do not get offended if you are sprayed with Lysol when you walk in the door and expect to wear mask, gloves and a fashionable yellow hospital gown. Hey...it is what it is!

I have to give kudos to Medical City Dallas and Texas Oncology! They were waiting for William in the ER yesterday and immediately took him to an isolated area. While doing paperwork, they had someone sterilizing a room for him. They quickly pulled blood and started testing for infections and had his chest x-rays done in a flash. Great job!

June 6
Day +141

Please pray for William. He passed out this morning and hit the floor hard! While unconscious, he started having convulsions. When he came to, he had a really bad headache and didn't have enough strength to get himself up. He was taken by ambulance to Medical City. They have pulled blood and are running tests. He is running a small fever and they are going to admit him. His doctor said his blood numbers are low, but not low enough to warrant concern "at this point." William has been having a lot of problems with his hemorrhoids again, and every time his platelets drop they start bleeding heavily and hurting again. His doctor said it appears a blood vessel has burst in one of them, and that he passed out from the pain. The plan for now is to keep him in the hospital on IV pain meds, and on Monday he will undergo some more tests. They are waiting for Monday because they want a stem cell/surgeon specialist to do his exam. Once we know the results of the tests, we have to confer with MD Anderson to determine the best treatment. Keep praying for him, he is still hurting but at least resting for now.

Ironically, today is one year since he was diagnosed! This day last year he was taken to the hospital with heart attack symptoms. While trying to diagnose a heart attack, they found his white cells were "funny shaped and out of whack." Very late into the evening they did a bone marrow biopsy. It was past 10:00 p.m. before they actually mentioned the word *leukemia*. I think they already knew, they just weren't saying it. I held on to a scrap of hope that it wouldn't be leukemia, that the biopsy would lead them to another diagnosis, but as you all know the results came back from the biopsy and confirmed a very aggressive cancer. His marrow was over 80% cancer, and the cancer was also in his central nervous system, on its way to his brain.

One year ago today, I did not even know that leukemia was a cancer. I knew it was bad, every parent's fear, but I did not know it was a blood cancer. I put it together when I entered his hospital room and saw the sign on the wall "Hematology Oncology" but still, my mind was looking for a way out. I thought maybe this was the only room they had available. The social worker came and said she needed permission to apply for disability for him. I couldn't think! WHY would William need disability? I gathered enough sense to tell her to go ahead. When I went back to his room, the doctor was waiting for me, three of them actually. They had the results, and it was a very nasty leukemia. Dr. Rutherford was his lead doctor and she told me, "He's a rare bird, this one. We are starting treatment right away. He is *very sick*."

This past year has been both a nightmare and a blessing. I have seen things that parents should not have to witness. I have seen side effects of treatments that are so inhumane you begin to question your decision to go through with it. I have felt my heart literally ache inside my chest with every beat. I have had to sit down with my son and discuss his final wishes, and plan his funeral with him because there was a very good chance he wasn't going to live. I had to learn to never lose my composure in front of him because I didn't want to scare him. I learned to cry silently while pushing his wheelchair. I had to practice asking the tough questions so I wouldn't break down crying in front of him. I have found strength I did not know was there.

Through the worst, I have also seen the best of people. I have made new friends, fellow cancer moms who have stood by me and held me up when I was physically unable to hold myself up. Family and friends who jumped in, organized blood drives, bone marrow drives, went grocery shopping, cooked meals, cleaned my house. They sprang into action for me while I walked around in a stupor. My mailbox filled with cards of hope and also financial gifts to help with food, gas, parking and the many extra expenses we would incur. I would not have made it without the help and encouragement from you all!

My faith has been stretched in ways I can't even begin to describe. "Faith is the substance of things hoped for, the confidence of things not seen." Even on the hardest days I held strong to my God because He was my only hope. When Jacob struggled with the Angel, he wouldn't let go until he was blessed. On the hardest, darkest days I told God I wasn't letting go until He healed him. Sometimes faith and hope are all you have, and all you need. One year later, and William is back in the hospital. Our fight is not over, and I am not letting go!

> *Comment 23: Sending many many, many prayers for William and mom too.. I know how hard it is to hear those words I passed out in the ER when they told me that my daughter had cancer... its tough ! Sending you lots of love and prayers ..*

> *Comment 55: Praying! I remember having the same feelings when my son was first diagnosed. Did not know that hematology treated leukemia so I felt a sense of relief until I saw the oncology part of it. Deep down I knew it was leukemia but was in denial til the official test results came in. Been a roller coaster ride ever since!*

> *Comment 64: Amy I am sorry William is going*

through this. I was concerned when you said they was taking his catheter out because when it comes to transplant it can sometimes throw you a curve. God has got this just try and stay calm and breath. As I read you post I remember having the same feelings. I felt so guilty because it would go through my mine that I brought Katie in this world and if I hadn't she wouldn't be suffering. But I wouldn't take a million dollars for the time I have had with her and the time I am going to have because of my savior Jesus Christ. Keep us posted. God Bless you and William and I will continue to pray.

Comment 87: Praying for you. You are amazing woman and I understand the strength that only God can give you through this. My mom has been in a 2 1/2 year fight and I am her warrior too!! It is a tough job but she is amazing and God has provided so many blessings even in the midst of the really hard down times. Continue to lean on him and your friends. You are both in my thoughts and prayers.

June 7
Day +142

Because William has the flu, he cannot be put on the floor with other transplant patients because it will put them at risk, so they put him on the Oncology floor. I walked toward his room, seeing those Chemotherapy and Oncology signs, and I was mentally pulled back to when he was diagnosed. I kept seeing the signs, and saying, "No, this isn't right, he doesn't have cancer!" I just cried. Even though I know he doesn't have cancer anymore, just seeing him on this floor brings up emotions I can't bear to feel.

June 9
Day +144

William finally saw the specialist this evening. His counts are too low to do any invasive exams or run a scope. It would put him in a very serious situation and the benefits don't outweigh the dangers. They need his white cells, red blood cells and platelets to come up, and rest is a key factor to that happening. The body heals when you sleep, so he needs a lot of sleep right now! They are keeping him comfortable and resting well, and the stem cell doctor and specialist are going to be closely watching him and monitoring his progress, symptoms and labs over the next several days. He is showing some possible GVHD symptoms in his eyes so this will also be very closely watched. At this point they are planning for him to remain in the hospital for a few more days until his labs stabilize and his symptoms subside.

June 14
Day +149

William was released a couple of days ago. At his follow-up appointment today he needed platelets and magnesium. His doctor said he just doesn't quite understand why his blood numbers are not improving. The medicine for the CMV that he took back in February started the downward spiral in his numbers. He has been off the medicine since March, but just can't seem to recover. Dr. Vance even suggested "something funny" was going on, but his last bone marrow biopsy looks really good. He said he wants to try to give him a series of IV immune globulin (IVIG) to see if it helps boost his numbers. It doesn't always work but he feels William is a good candidate to try it since he has had CMV and the flu. It will be done over ten weeks and should help boost his overall immune system. There's no guarantee but it's worth a try.

June 20
Day +155

William is getting platelets again today. His other labs are holding steady but not coming up. The doctor is waiting on insurance approval to start the IVIG. Hopefully they will approve it quickly, but I kind of worry about it. If we don't have an answer by Monday I guess I will have to get on the phone and do a little begging!

I have been quarantined away from William for several days now. Both James and Abbey have been sick with a viral upper respiratory infection and they were so kind to share their germs with me, so now I am sick too. It may be another week before I get to see him but I know Mom and Dad are taking good care of him.

June 25
Day +160

William is very downhearted right now. He went for labs and yet again his platelets are low. He is getting a transfusion. I talked to him on the phone (I am still isolated from him) and he said he feels as if he is never going to get over this; that he is never going to be able to make any plans or have a future! I can't begin to understand how he feels! William has been sick for over a year - that has to be so hard on him emotionally. Please pray, and pray hard for his blood numbers to jump up and stay up.

The stitches holding his chest catheter in are coming loose too. He may end up having to have it removed, but if so his doctor might put a PICC line back in. The PICC is the one that he used to have, inserted in the arm. It is less maintenance than the CVC (the chest catheter) but still allows for easier blood draws and transfusions without having to "stick" him each time or run an IV. Of course, if his blood numbers come up and stay up, he won't need the PICC or the CVC, and that would be the best option.

July 3
Day +168

William's blood numbers are still just crazy! He had to get a platelet transfusion earlier in the week, and narrowly missed getting red blood today. His hemoglobin dropped under 10. Personally, I would have transfused, but he was really glad they didn't. I reminded him to take it easy and be extra careful this weekend. He goes back on Monday for a recheck. I spoke with his stem cell doctor at MD Anderson, and they really aren't overly concerned at this point. He will be back there in two weeks for several tests on his lungs, heart and bones and another bone marrow biopsy, so we are all hoping one of these tests will shed some light on what might be going on. And there is always the fact that some people just take longer to recover. That may be the case with William.

I went to Carter Blood Care yesterday and donated blood. Friends, they are in serious need! I got there shortly after noon and I was only the *second* donation of the day. Summer is tough on all blood centers. Please remember that donated blood products continue to keep William alive, and all cancer patients rely on them to live. Please, please, please take 30 minutes out of your day and give blood! I hate needles too, but I remind myself what William has been through, and if he can go through all that, I can handle one little needle prick in the arm! So please, if you can, go out there and give blood and save a life today!

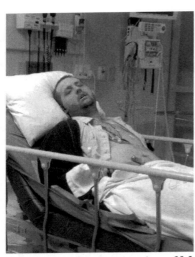

July 5
Day +170

So we are back in the ER! God give me the strength and patience NOT to slap this rude charge nurse, or at least good friends to help me post bail if I do!

Update: William is in a room now. We have no idea at this point how long he will stay in the hospital. He will be getting two units of blood and platelets this evening. He wasn't feeling well earlier and took a nap. When he woke up he was lying in a pool of blood. We do not really know if it is a burst hemorrhoid or what, but he is losing a lot of blood! This could be transplant related or some residual effects from the seven months of harsh chemo he had to take in order to get into and stay in remission for his transplant. The seven months of chemo just damaged his body so badly! Some of the issues may heal in time but some will not. His oxygen level was dropping pretty low so they did x-ray his chest again, looking for pneumonia. They are also entertaining the possibility of a relapse, so they are looking for evidence of that as well.

Tomorrow he will see the stem cell doctor and they will come up with a plan. Right now he will get blood and pain meds to keep him as comfortable as possible for the time being.

Luckily I didn't have to go to jail for assault! ☺ I have to say once we got him to his room; the nurses on the floor were fantastic! They more than made up for the one bad apple down in the ER. But I am still filing a complaint tomorrow with her supervisor.

Right now I am just praying for a restful night for William, and for some clear direction in the morning once he sees the stem cell doctor and we have his tests results back.

> *Comment 10: Praying he gets better soon. And I am sure if needed we can come up with your bail $!!!*

> *Comment 17: I'll post bail...go for it...I'll even come help you...and bring my handcuffs, but not for you...lol....I have more people praying..He has to keep up his courage and good thoughts...this will pass...do not give up...keep fighting.*

> *Comment 30: Aw, that's horrible. Feel better & hope her shift ends SOON!!*

*Comment 33: Call me and I'll come bail you out...
and take you for a drink before we go back to
teach her a lesson. Love ya!:-)*

*Comment 50: I'm sorry to hear that William is
back in the ER. We continue to pray for him. It's
unfortunate (regarding the nurse) that they can't
teach kindness in school. If you land in jail, I'll chip
in for your bail! Hang in there.*

July 6
Day +171

William received blood and platelets throughout the night and his numbers are up for now. The stem cell doctor examined him this morning and is addressing some of his complications but is calling in a specialist to address the bleeding from his rectum. Today he wants William to rest. He has lost a lot of blood in the last few days and his body needs recovery time and rest.

The x-rays from the ER showed nothing out of the ordinary in William's lungs or spleen. This is incredibly comforting because an enlarged spleen could signify a relapse, but thank God we don't have to entertain that possibility anymore!

So lots of rest for today and more doctors tomorrow. Once everyone has seen him we should have a game plan on how to move forward. Being he is not quite six months post transplant, he is still on immunosuppressive medicines and his labs are very unstable they are taking every possible caution with him. All of the doctors are consulting with the stem cell doctor to make sure the benefits outweigh the risks in every possible treatment plan.

July 8
Day +173

William is going to undergo surgery tomorrow. He has been losing blood since Saturday and has an abscess in his colon. The surgeon believes it is very possibly GVHD related. The doctors have been monitoring his blood loss every eight hours since he was admitted on Saturday. They will give him extra platelets today to help raise his counts before surgery.

This is a very serious condition because of his low blood and platelet counts, and because he is neutropenic as well. However it is more dangerous not to address this now. It will not get better without intervention and the risk of further infection is just too great. Please, lots of prayers for a smooth and uneventful surgery, and complete and fast healing.

Right now he is on very strong IV pain meds and sleeping most of the time, but his doctor said that is the best thing he can do right now for his body.

July 9
Day +174

10:34 a.m.: William's surgery has had to put be on hold. His platelets are too low and there are *no compatible platelets* in the entire Dallas region! William *has to have* type-specific platelets or he has terrible reactions. Please, if you are A+ blood type, ask your boss/supervisor/HR person if you can leave work and go donate platelets. It will take two hours to donate. Go to Carter Blood Care to donate, whichever donation center is nearest to you. He is also running a fever now!

12:55 p.m.: The hospital put out a critical need request and a bag of platelets were brought over from Bedford. William is scheduled for surgery at 5:00 p.m. today. The infection is spreading and he is running a fever. His blood pressure has dropped to 71/39! They have started IV antibiotics to help control the infection, but the surgery is critical! Please keep donating those platelets! He will need several units in the days ahead. All blood centers are critically low right now and there are many people just like William in need. Trust me, every donation counts. There are lots of frantic moms out there praying for blood and platelets. I speak for all of them when I say thank you! I will keep you posted through the day. Keep donating, keep

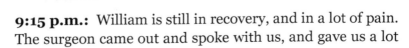

praying, and thank you...thank you!

5:12 p.m.: He is off to surgery, with another bag of platelets waiting on him in the operating room. His blood pressure came up to the safe zone so we have a green light. They just gave him the "lights out" medicine.

9:15 p.m.: William is still in recovery, and in a lot of pain. The surgeon came out and spoke with us, and gave us a lot of technical explanation which honestly I barely remember. Here is what I do remember: William is going be ok! It wasn't as bad as the surgeon had feared. The infection has cleared and he did not see any signs of active GVHD. We had some scary moments today, at one point William's blood pressure dropped to 71/39. But right now, I just keep hearing the surgeon saying "He is going to be just fine!"

I honestly cannot begin to express how thankful I am for all your support! I have gone from crying in one minute because I was so full of gratitude, to laughing in the next minute because I was so happy! Pictures, posts and texts have been coming from all over the country. Folks were donating at their local blood centers in William's honor, and Carter Blood Care in Mesquite was packed today.

William is going to continue to need platelets for a long time. During all this mess we also found the answer as to why his platelets have been so low. In his last bone marrow biopsy, the immature platelets count was markedly low, so his new marrow is slow to make platelets. His doctor suspects he will need platelet support for at least six more months, possibly as long as a year. But it answers the question as to *why*. Knowing he will continue to need transfusions, we had to address his CVC (chest catheter). It had come unstitched and was coming out so they removed it and put a PICC line in. The PICC is the same thing, but different. It is still a catheter, but it has two lumens instead of three and it is inserted into his arm and the catheter line runs into his heart like the other one did. But the PICC line is easier to maintain, easier to shower with, easier for bandage changes and still allows easy access for blood draws and transfusions or IV's.

Wow, what a day! I am so relieved, and again I just can't thank y'all enough for all your wonderful help, prayers, support, everything! You're all just amazing!

> *Comment 3: I donated platelets today and I 'm scheduled again in August. I'll try to see that the platelets go to him if possible.*

> *Comment 4: What wonderful news! Hundreds of us are going to go to sleep tonight with great relief in our hearts knowing William is doing better!*

> *Comment 10: God is always with William, that much is evident.*

> *Comment 20: Amy- Over on Timothy's page (Timothy's Leukemia Journey) an amazing lady, Tiffany, donated platelets today after I posted a request! She did it for William!!!! Continuing to send our love & Prayers!*

> *Comment 22: I pray rest so profoundly over you . May you sleep like a baby without a sorry in the world. Gods on duty He does not sleep. Rest. Praises and Glory to Jesus.*

> *Comment 39: Gracias Diosito!!! Thank God!!!*

> *Comment 43: This brought tears to my eyes I'm so happy William is going to be ok. He is a very strong young man. Thank you God for being with him.*

Comment 49: Praising God for William and all of your family. You all mean so much to me. Love you all.

July 10

Day +175

William is doing well. He was awake and alert most of the day. He is still in a lot of pain, but he is requiring less pain medicine than in the last several days. His blood pressure has remained stable in the safe zone all day, and no fever. They are keeping him on IV antibiotics just to make sure all infection is gone. Normally he hates being in the hospital but today he told me he was glad he was there, and doesn't feel ready to go home. I don't believe I have ever heard those words come out of his mouth! Now he just needs to eat. It's been two or three days now since he has.

Comment 9: I am so grateful to God to hear this news. I've checked for updates all day. Eat, William! (In my teacher voice)

Comment 16: William eat (the cop's voice). Do I need to call Gary in on this. Wink. Love you

Comment 27: Miracles do happen and I thank God for letting you be one of his miracles , I know he is watching over you!

July 12

Day +177

Sometimes the journey back to wellness is one step forward, and TWO steps back! Today is one of those days. The antibiotic used to clear William's original infection has led to him getting CDIFF. CDIFF is a bacterial infection in your colon (usually brought on by using a lot of antibiotics). The interesting thing is that it is caused by antibiotics and is treated with antibiotics. So today he starts new antibiotics. His doctor hopes to be able to send him home on Monday, but we'll see.

Talk about frustrating! William told me the other day he feels like he will never get better. It is so hard to try to stay positive all the time while he is getting beat down at every turn. You can really only say, "Just get over this hurdle then you can get back on the road to recovery" so many times before it loses its effectiveness. I know that eventually he really WILL hit that point where he is recovering and getting stronger but I sure wish I knew for certain when that was going to happen. Two years seems to be the magic number for most transplant survivors, so I told him yesterday to put that number in his mind. This way he doesn't get so discouraged, and he is already six months into it at this point. I don't know if it helped him any, but it's kind of all I have right now.

He's been through so much and he has handled it so well! I am so very proud of him! My mom has always told us that the pendulum swings both directions, and as far as it swings on the negative side will be as far as it swings on the positive side. Let me just say, I am SO ready for his pendulum to change directions!

> *Comment 4: I'm sorry you're having all the roller coasters. It was roughly two years before i got stronger. Don't lose hope William!!!!*

> *Comment 10: My son is almost 4 years post transplant. Don't give up. We also went through a*

lot of hurdles in the first year, thinking it will never end or see the end of the tunnel. My son is now doing well, back to all the normal things that a 9year old boy should be doing. I will pray for his peace of mind and most especially his health!

Comment 11: My mom has had several bouts of CDIFF in the last two years. Its no fun at all.. Even had to have a special made just for her to try and get rid of it. The medicine was $3000. Had to fight insurance to pay for it

Comment 14: You'll get there William. It took Daniela over a year to get better. She had a lots of back steps too. Don't give up, think positive, even if it's hard sometimes.

Comment 17: Hang in there William. I understand all too well how these setbacks make you feel. BUT this too shall pass! It WILL get better! Look how far you have come since you were first diagnosed. May God give you strength & patience William~~~ they're happy and better days ahead! We will still be right here for you all~ praying!

Comment 21: My daughter went through similar feelings after her bmt. It was hardest right around the 6 month part. She had finally started feeling better, and just like William, ugly side effects from the chemo and radiation kicked in. Tell him to hang in there. He WILL get better. It may take a little more time, but he will get there. So will you.

Comment 24: I don't know you, but I am praying your family and I have an appointment to give platelets next Saturday. Don't give up

July 13
Day +178

I do have better news to share today. William is stronger, and he finally ate an actual meal. We talked for a bit and I read your encouraging comments from yesterday to him. We discussed keeping two years as a goal to return to wellness, and in the meantime taking baby steps to get there. This way it won't be so discouraging every time he hits a bump in the road. He told me some of his long term plans and we talked about how to set small goals to help him achieve the big ones, and still allow for all his medical appointments, numerous transfusions and the occasional hospital stay.

His doctor hopes to send him home tomorrow so he can rest up and make the trip back to Houston for his six month post transplant checkup at the end of this week. Thank you all so much for your positive comments, messages and texts, and for keeping William and my entire family in your prayers!

Comment 9: My daughter is 2 yrs post transplant and yes 2 years is a good goal! My baby is finally doing well and back at school. Hang in there!!

Comment 12: Proud of you William. Praying for you every day. We're just going to take baby steps now.

Comment 17: I'm so proud of you for eating, William, as well as encouraged about you making short-term and long-term goals. I know this has been discouraging, but it seems as if it's just part of your fight. Who knew that when I met you, when you were a little boy, you would become such a fighter and encouragement to me? Well, God knew. We are all in His hands and His plans for us. I'm glad I didn't have to come use my teacher-voice with you or make you "turn your bus." (We might be the only ones who know what I'm talking about.) Keep up your hopes, and fight on. Never, never, never give up. Love you, Amy, too.

Comment 20: It is an honor to be a part of the WILLIAM TEAM

July 16
Day +181

Mark your calendar for July 29. My friend Kendra has set up a blood drive at Mockingbird Station from 9:00 a.m.-4:00 p.m. I plan to be there all day so if you live local, please come by and say hi (and leave a pint of blood if you can). Krispy Kreme is donating donuts for everyone and my sister-in-law is making up some of her fabulous brownies. I will also have swab kits on hand if you want to join the bone marrow registry.

William is back home and getting ready to go back to Houston to see his MDA team tomorrow for his six month post transplant checkup and tests. He will have another bone marrow biopsy on Friday. Today he is seeing his local doctor to make sure his blood and platelet levels are okay for the trip.

July 17
Day +182

William is at MD Anderson with my mom and dad. He met with his stem cell doctor, Dr. Champlin, this afternoon. After a few questions, they felt that he was showing signs that his GVHD of the gut was returning. They canceled all scheduled tests, including his bone marrow biopsy and scheduled him for an endoscopy and biopsy of the upper GI tract tomorrow at 11:00 a.m.

This evening they are giving him platelets to raise his levels to the safe zone to have the endoscopy/biopsy. This will confirm or rule out GVHD, and of course if it comes back positive they will treat him appropriately. Mom said they had a sense of urgency to get this done since GVHD of the gut can be fatal if left untreated. I am not sure how soon we will have test results, or if they will have to stay in Houston until results are in. It's all up in the air right now. His regular six month tests have been postponed until next month. They said right now, this is more urgent.

Hopefully we will have the results very soon so we know what to expect moving forward. I will post an update once we know, but I surely would covet your prayers while we wait.

July 18
Day +183

William and my parents are on the way home. William is very tired and sore. The surgeon did find that his stomach is inflamed so they did a biopsy. We will not have those results for several days. Since he has a history of GVHD in

288

his GI tract, I expect the biopsy to come back positive, but I have been wrong before, so we will wait for the professionals to diagnose him!

Don't forget the blood drive on July 29. Please come by if you can. I will be there all day. If you gave platelets last week, you may be eligible to donate whole blood, but check with Carter Blood Care. If you are not eligible to donate you can still come by and say hi. Hugs and donuts are free, and we'll have plenty of both.

July 24
Day +189

Well color me wrong! William's biopsy came back negative for GVHD in his stomach. We don't know what is causing the inflammation in his stomach, but we know it isn't GVHD. He goes back to MD Anderson next month to take the tests he missed last week and we will revisit the stomach issue with his stem cell doctor at that time. He is also being monitored by his local stem cell doctor.

July 29
Day +194

Today was awesome! The blood drive was a great success! We ended up with 34 blood donations and 21 people signed up for the bone marrow registry. William was able to stop by for just a few minutes. He has been very weak and tired, so he was only able to stay for about five minutes before having to leave. I had time to sit down and talk with almost every donor, and met some incredible folks today. I feel really blessed.

This evening William began to feel light headed and "not right" so he is in the ER right now having his blood numbers checked. He was low on platelets last week so I am sure he needs a transfusion now, and possibly some magnesium. He is in an isolated area right now. Mom and Dad are with him and we are waiting on lab results. I will keep you posted once I know something. Thank you to everyone who donated today, and those who tried but weren't able to. Each donation will save up to three lives. And for everyone that signed up for the bone marrow registry. I am so proud of all of you and thankful for the time I was able to spend with you today.

8:25 p.m.: William's platelets and hemoglobin levels are both low, and he is bleeding at his surgery site. The bleeding has gotten heavier as the day progressed, probably from the low platelets. They have decided it would be in his best interest to admit him to the hospital so they can carefully monitor his bleeding and give him blood and platelet transfusions. The ER doctor noticed his coloring was gray too, so she just felt it was too risky to send him home.

July 31
Day +196

William gets to come home today. Once his platelets were back up in a safe zone, the bleeding stopped. I spoke with the surgeon this morning and I asked him if the bleeding was directly related to the low platelets. He believes it is. He is going to speak with both stem cell doctors and stress the importance of raising William's platelet transfusion threshold to help avoid future bleeding issues.

I spoke with William on the phone this morning and he

sounds much stronger! He said once he got the platelets and magnesium he felt better and stronger. I told him he really needs two blood checks a week until his platelets get higher and are more predictable. He said, "Mom I am very predictable! I go into the hospital every two weeks like clockwork!"

Yeah, he's getting back to normal!

August 6
Day +202

William has been sleeping a lot, and I mean A LOT over the last few days. This used to concern me, but not so much anymore. I have noticed that when he sleeps a long time, he wakes up stronger than before. I have come to the conclusion that his body is healing when he goes through those thirty-hour sleep cycles, and we just need to let his body work.

He ended up needing platelets again yesterday at his blood checkup appointment. They were very low again. I spoke with his surgeon and his stem cell doctor and we have all decided it is in William's best interest to keep doing two lab checks a week for right now. Normally the hospital will not transfuse until a patient's platelet level drops to 15, but I asked if we could raise that benchmark for William since he has a history of open bleeding at his surgery site when his platelets drop. We can't keep running him to the ER every two weeks when it could be prevented by just transfusing before he gets so critically low. Both doctors agree that's the best plan of action right now, so they are watching closely to see where to set his benchmarks. Right now, they will transfuse at 23, and if he still bleeds at 23 they will raise it to 30. I am glad the doctors are so easy to talk to, and are accommodating of my questions, concerns and suggestions.

We head back to Houston in a week and a half to make up the six month tests he had to miss last month. They cancelled some of his tests so they could do the endoscopy/biopsy so now we need to make them up. We will get updated information on his heart and lung damage and do another bone marrow biopsy. I always get nervous over those. So much rides on those results.

August 9
Day +205

Please say a prayer for William. He is running a low fever, abdominal cramping and vomiting. He has thrown up all of his medicines. We are closely watching and waiting to see if we need to take him to the ER. I am seriously praying it's just a stomach bug and not anything more serious.

August 10
Day +206

Dad took William to the hospital last night about 8:30 p.m. His fever spiked and vomiting was out of control. They gave him IV meds and did an abdominal scan. The scan was normal, which helped rule out some underlying problems. His symptoms are in line with a pretty bad stomach virus. For most of us, something like this isn't a major ordeal, but to an immunosuppressive person it can be. They were able to give him meds to stop the vomiting and something for the cramping. He wasn't able to take his medicines yesterday, which is a big concern! He and Daddy left the hospital around 3:00 a.m., so today they are resting. William is still very sore and nauseated. He took his 6:00 a.m. meds and so far has held them down.

August 11
Day +207

Have you ever felt like you get up only to be slapped back down? Well I got a call from the ER nurse this afternoon. When William went to the ER Saturday night, they ran blood cultures. This is a common practice for transplant patients. One of his cultures is showing an infection. Early indications are a staph infection, but we will know for sure by tomorrow. They have started treating him with Vancomycin, but may change that depending on what grows in the cultures. But he will be going back to the outpatient infusion clinic every day this week except Thursday. So he had not only a stomach virus, but also a secondary infection. He was pretty downhearted to hear he had another infection but he was glad the treatment could be done outpatient.

I am to the point now that when my phone rings and I see the prefix numbers for either Medical City or MD Anderson, I take a deep breath and brace myself before answering! This poor kid needs a break! I keep reminding myself "two years, two years, you know it may take two years for his body to recover." I think at the end of that two year period we are going to need a very long vacation! Any suggestions where we should go?

Comment 1: Far away! I know it's hard but never

forget it's not forever. God knows the plan, we just have to keep looking to Him. All things work together for good. We're grateful they discovered it now. Blessings to William and the family.

Comment 9: I can't imagine how tired all of you are of this, and how scary it must be when they call. Praying that this infection will also get beaten right away. As for a vacation, maybe some place quiet and serene, without a lot of people around?

Comment 11: Destin Florida. Better yet, Newport, Rhode Island.

Comment 13: Cozumel Mexico!!! All inclusive resort

Comment 15: Mountain retreat with streams and calming walks!!! JUST BREATHE!!!! Cook simple and enjoy the beauty....that's what I want!!!!

Comment 34: Honey go to a beach

August 16
Day +212

William received a call today that his blood cultures are still growing and not responding to the Vancomycin. The infection started in his PICC line so they removed it yesterday. He did another round of antibiotics today through a regular IV and will do another round tomorrow through an IV. On Monday morning we are heading to MDA to do the six month post transplant tests that had to be postponed last month. Plus he will have a new PICC line inserted.

William is tired. He is tired of being sick. He is not in a good emotional state right now. When we see his stem cell doctor at MDA, we really need to have a long talk. William doesn't seem to be getting better; he seems to be getting worse. I have a nagging feeling that something just isn't right. Maybe one of the tests will reveal something. I don't know. I just know we need to find out what's happening and address it. Please pray with me that whatever is going on will be brought to light, so that he can finally get back on the road to recovery! And please pray for strength for William as he continues to take this physical and emotional beating.

August 19
Day +215

We are back from MDA. We are both very tired! William and I left the hospital after midnight last night, and we're back at 6:00 this morning for more tests. Then we headed home. It was a good trip, and we were able to talk with his stem cell doctor about our concerns. William has been afraid his transplant didn't work, and afraid he was going to need a second one. Dr. Champlin was able to reassure us that when they do a bone marrow biopsy, they are looking for much more than just cancer cells, and absolutely nothing has come up in the last several of William's biopsies that would raise a red flag.

Dr. Champlin is convinced that what has happened is that when a patient goes through long term chemo, and high doses of it, the bone marrow "environment" sustains a lot of damage and it takes longer to rebound. He feels this is what is going on with William. William's immune globulin has also been low, so he needs IVIG (IV administered

Immune Globulin). He feels this will give William's immune system a substantial boost and help bring his platelet count up. Now here is the problem, IVIG is upwards of $20,000 a bag! He needs one bag a month for the next year. That's $240,000! So we need insurance to approve this.

For those who have been on this journey with us for awhile, you will remember the issues getting the transplant approved. I am gearing up for another fight, so I need to ask your prayers that they will just approve it quickly. The faster they approve it, the sooner William will begin to feel better. This is important for both his physical and mental health.

It will be about a week before we have the biopsy results, and of course we nervously await those. We are still hoping, praying and believing for zero cancer!

August 22
Day +218

One of the ways cancer has changed me is my perception of time. I had always taken it for granted, assuming I had all the time in the world to do anything I wanted. But one day, I stood next to a hospital bed, looking at my son in complete disbelief as a team of doctors gathered around his bed. "He has leukemia, he is very sick! The cancer has already penetrated his central nervous system, and on its way to his brain. We need to start chemo right away or he will die within a couple of days."

In one way, time stopped. In another way the clock started ticking louder than ever! It was my first realization that I might lose him. Once we found out how aggressive his cancer actually was, time became a very precious commodity! Some nights in the hospital we would stay up late and talk. I would be so sleepy, but he would hold my hand and ask me to stay awake and keep talking to him. Time was all we had, and for that moment we DID have it, so we had to make the most of it.

William's donor gave us the most precious gift of all; she gave us more time! Before his transplant, I could hear the clock ticking. William could *feel* it ticking away. He told me one night he could feel the chemo killing him; he was dying slowly with every dose. Back then, I could only look ahead one day at a time and sometimes only one minute at a time. Now that we are on the other side of the transplant I can look further ahead again. I set my time by bone marrow biopsies now. They run about two months apart. As each one approaches, panic raises up inside me. I know so much hinges on those results!

I got a call yesterday from MD Anderson. The preliminary results from Tuesday's biopsy are in. Once again, we can breathe a sigh of relief. The preliminary results show no leukemia cells! His next biopsy is scheduled for October 20, and I am sure I will go through the panic as it gets closer. But for now, I have time again! My clock is re-set and I am focusing on spending less time on my computer, Kindle and phone and spending more time with the things that really matter...my family!

August 23
Day +219

I spoke with William's insurance case manager yesterday, and she has already approved the IVIG for MD Anderson! She asked me to have Medical City Dallas also submit a request for it so William could get it at either location. She will be looking for the request and approve it right away! His case manager has been a very big help for us through the last several months.

William is scheduled to get his first dose this coming Wednesday. I have emotions running through me that I can't quite find the words to express. Joy, anticipation, relief! So much relief! William's damaged body has worked so hard to recover, but there is just so much to repair! He has needed this boost for so long. Now his body and his medication can work in unison to repair and rebuild.

He will never return to the same life he had before. The chemo left some of his organs permanently damaged, and he will have certain limitations that will stay with him for the rest of his life. But he will learn to adapt to those changes and limitations; he will learn a new normal and he WILL regain his life!

With this approval, we are closing a very dark chapter in his life, and opening a new, brighter one. A new chapter full of hope and promise! Hope that his cancer stays in remission and never returns. Hope that his body will quickly rebound and his strength will return. Hope that he will continue to grow and mature into the future God has in store for him. And most of all promise! Promise that through it all, we were able to bear witness that NOTHING is too wonderful for The Lord!

AFTERWARD

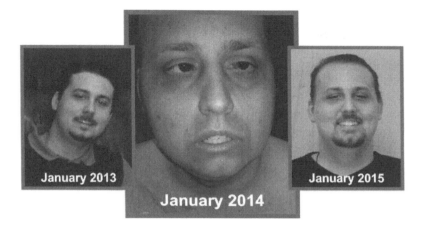

January 2013

January 2014

January 2015

Our journey is not over, it continues day by day. It is strange that I have peace, but I do not think I will ever BE at peace. The fear of a relapse will always be at the back of my mind. Some of the chemos used to treat leukemia can actually *cause* leukemia. One of the side effects of Doxorubicin, otherwise known as the "Red Devil" is leukemia. William took high doses of this chemo, and therefore increases his chance of relapsing. I know our lives will never be the same as they were before William's diagnosis. You can look at the before cancer and after treatment pictures of William and see how he has changed physically. You can see the devastating toll chemo has taken on him. His lungs function like that of a 70 year old, and his heart of a 67 year old. I wonder how many years have been cut from his life. With every cold, every illness I am thrown back to the reality of William's delicate health and the possibility that his cancer has returned. Cancer changes you. While everyone's cancer experience is different, one thing is the same of everyone, both patient and caregiver: when you come out of this journey, you will be different than you were when you began it.

I have learned a lot as I have helped my son fight his way through cancer and recovery. I want to share some of my "take-aways" from this experience to help you if you or someone you know ever ends up in a similar situation.

- Several well-meaning people told me "Oh, it's Leukemia, thank God! That's the GOOD cancer." I know they were trying to comfort me but after walking this journey, let me be the first to say this, "There is no such thing as a GOOD cancer!" *Stop saying that!* All cancer can kill! I almost buried my son because of the "good" cancer! All cancer brings chemo, radiation, surgery, or any combination of the three. It's ALL BAD! Treatable or not, it's all bad! If you want to offer words of encouragement, just put your arms around my neck, hug me while I cry, and say you are there for me. Tell me you have faith he will beat it! Just say "This sucks and I wish I could fix it." That's all I need.

- Accept the help that is offered to you. You are going to run out of milk and toilet paper. If a friend calls and offers to go shopping for you, accept it. You will not have the energy to cook, grocery shop, make phone calls, clean your house, pay your bills or any of the regular daily things you do. If you are looking for a way to help a friend with cancer please consider some of these ways to help. For nearly a week after William's diagnosis, I didn't eat anything but my other children and my husband still needed to eat. Family and neighbors fed them for me. It was a huge help! Some days I just gave James and Abbey Oreos for breakfast because it was easy and no thinking was required. I asked a group of cancer moms what were the most meaningful ways people helped them after their child's diagnosis, and here were their responses:

o Grocery shop for them

o Cook for them and deliver it in throw-away containers so they don't have to worry about cleaning and returning your dish.

o Clean their house or pay someone to do it, even a one-time clean is an amazing help.

o Cut their grass, rake leaves, clean gutters, and/or winterize the pipes and plants (season depending).

o Walk their dog(s) on a schedule.

o Gift cards for groceries, gas and local restaurants are very helpful. Hospital parking is incredibly expensive too, cash for parking, coffee and lunch at the hospital is also appreciated.

o If it's a co-worker, ask HR if you and fellow employees can donate some of your sick or vacation time so the person can be off work and not lose pay (especially important for single moms). Then rally up the troops to pitch in.

o Host a fundraiser. Cancer is incredibly expensive, even with insurance. There are thousands upon thousands of dollars of added expenses that insurance will not cover. Financial gifts of any, and every amount help!

o Remember the other children. Sometimes the siblings get lost because the sick child gets all the attention and gifts. Offer to sit with the sick child so the parents can take the other kids out for ice cream once in awhile.

o Pick up siblings from school.

o Come visit me at the hospital, and bring food. Hospital food is usually terrible and expensive!

o Don't ask me "What can I do for you?" Honestly, I am in such a stupor that I can't even think to tell you what I need! Don't ask, just pick something and DO!

• Paperwork is a nightmare! You will get piles of papers thrown at you from all directions. You will be writing notes and taking phone numbers on scraps of papers, envelopes and napkins. Save everything! As soon as you throw something away, you will need it and you will waste hours looking for it. Get a box, and throw every scrap of paper in the box. This way when you need something, you have one box to search instead of thirty places around your house. If you have time to create a file system, that works too. The goal is just to keep all papers in one place. If you are going to be filing for any type of grants or aid, you need to gather bank statements, birth certificate, driver's license, medical records, social security cards, tax returns and pay stubs. I even had to show William's voter registration card. Some other paperwork you may need to gather, if it applies, would be your spouse's death certificate, divorce decree, child support orders and statements, US passport, INS documentation, life insurance policies, car titles, mortgage statements, stocks/bonds or other securities and/or trusts, oil lease royalties or any other assets recently transferred or not included on your tax return. These are just some of the papers you will need to gather. Each entity will have its own specific list of required documentation. I put all the papers in a file and carried them everywhere with me. I would get phone calls while at the hospital, and the papers would be at home. It caused delays in processing so I learned to bring everything with me, until all grants and aids were filed and we had the approvals. Another helpful tip is when dealing with Social Security, they will not accept copies. All documents have to be original. This becomes an issue of you get your bank statements online or your paystubs are online only.

- **Financial help is out there!** Your best source for knowing all your financial aid options would be the hospital social worker. He/She usually has a list of local entities that offer help. In Texas, you can apply for a one-time grant up to $750 for Heroes for Children if the patient is under 21 and has a cancer diagnosis. The request must be submitted from a hospital social worker, and then they will email you a questionnaire to determine how much you can qualify for. Leukemia Texas also has a quarterly grant up to $1000, but the application must be filled out by a doctor and include a leukemia diagnosis. The social worker at the hospital is a wealth of information for discounts on hotels if you have to travel away from home. If your hospital doesn't automatically arrange for you to meet with the social worker, you can request it. Just ask your doctor or the charge nurse to contact the social worker for a meeting. Be sure to ask if the hospital has a financial aid program. With insurance or not, when your bills are in the million dollar range any financial aid is a help! Ask if the hospital offers parking vouchers. Parking fees are usually not reimbursed by insurance, and those fees can quickly add up!

- Trust your gut! If you feel something is wrong, voice it. Sometimes doctors will gloss over a symptom and dismiss it as normal. But if something isn't "sitting right" with you, do not accept that as an answer. I call it the Mom Radar. Embrace it, trust it! When I took William to the emergency room in October, I knew he needed blood. His local treating hospital said his hemoglobin wasn't low enough to transfuse, but I knew he had been taking the ARA-C chemo, and I knew from past experience that chemo caused his hemoglobin to drop into the 5 range. I argued with the doctor and he insisted William didn't need blood, even though his hemoglobin was only 8. I knew William wouldn't make it to the next doctor appointment. Within two days he ran low fever, and I took him to Houston to MD Anderson. When we got to the ER he wasn't even running a fever. They will tell you to bring them to the ER if the fever gets over 100.5, but I explained about his low hemoglobin and they didn't even question me. They drew blood and did chest x-rays and he needed four units of blood and had double pneumonia. He was admitted for an eight-day stay. If in your gut you feel like something is wrong, fight for your patient.   If you think he needs to have a test run, insist on it. I learned early on; when you are fighting for your loved one it's okay to get loud, and sometimes you just have to!

- A small victory is still a victory! Cancer is a beast, and the treatments are horrific! The chemo breaks the body down both physically and emotionally. You have to celebrate every positive, no matter how small. Every time they can get up and walk around, it's a victory! Every time they can eat, it's a victory! Going 24 hours without nausea meds, victory! Getting out of the wheelchair and using a cane, victory! This is not a short-term illness, and there are many setbacks along the way so staying positive is crucial for the mental health of the patient as well as the caregiver.

- It's okay to be angry! I felt guilty when I was angry, I felt like I wasn't exercising my faith enough. But it didn't change the fact I was angry. I read spiritual books, and that only made me feel worse. I know that my son's cancer didn't take God by surprise, but it sure did me! My perfect, wonderful world had come to an end. I finally realized that being angry is part of the grieving cycle. When I opened up and shared my feelings with other cancer moms I found out they were feeling the same way. I suggest you find a trusted friend, family member or professional counselor and share your grief. Find someone who will just listen. For those on the listening side, this is not the time to remind me that "God will never give you more than you can handle" or "everything happens for a reason." I know it sounds comforting, but when you are in the middle of the grieving cycle you need time to work through your emotions. Most of my fellow cancer moms found those two statements to be the most offensive "words of comfort" they were given. This is just a time to listen and let me cry and yell and ask WHY! More than likely, in time they will realize these statements to be true, but it takes time. Just be there, no advice, just listen!

- Never give up. The original diagnosis will send you into shock. You don't hear everything, and the mind tends to focus on the worse. Add to that the fact we all have a built in fear of cancer and it's a mental recipe for disaster! Percentages run through your head, survival rates, etc. In our case, we were given a good outlook in the beginning. But as William's treatment progressed, it became very grim. When his doctor looked down at the floor and shook his head, my heart dropped and I felt like I had just been given William's death sentence. My husband became the eternal optimist, and kept telling me don't give up, it isn't over! Don't focus on the treatment that didn't work, or how aggressive his cancer is. Focus on the hope that there are still more treatment options left. One will work! My husband kept telling me "It isn't over, don't give up!" Hearing the words kept me from focusing on the negative and looking for the positive. It is also important to never give up if you have to fight your insurance company. William's transplant was denied two times. We kept appealing, and kept fighting. Denial meant certain death, and that was not an option. I had already determined that if the insurance wasn't going to allow his transplant, I was going to raise the 1.2 million dollars for it. No matter what circumstances are thrown at you, keep fighting, and never give up!

- You will receive tons of unsolicited medical advice! Everyone will read the miracle cure on the Internet and tell you that you don't have to do this horrible chemo. You just need to stop treatments, and do this or that and you will be cured. Understand your friends and family mean well, and by all means discuss it with your doctor if you feel led to, but always follow your doctor's advice. I talked to William's doctor about medical marijuana, and they did offer it to William but he chose not to accept the prescription. It would not have cured his cancer, but it would have made the side effects of his treatment more tolerable. William wasn't comfortable taking it, and I honored his wishes. It is also important not to accept medications, herbal remedies, essential oils, vitamins or anything before you discuss it with your medical professional. At one point William was having terrible issues with his hemorrhoids. I had a prescription hemorrhoid cream left over from when I was pregnant, so without thinking I gave it to William to use. He had the sense to wait to ask his doctor about it, and thank goodness he did. There was a very serious drug interaction with one of his medications. Do not take it for granted that because it is herbal or "all natural" that is will be safe! Before you take any form of pill, cream, liquid or essential oil in any way, shape, form or fashion, ask your doctor.

- Caregivers need care too! Being a caregiver is one of the most difficult jobs in the world. Caregivers get so caught up in the needs of the patient they forget to take care of their own needs. This is fine for a short-term situation, but it will not work for a long-term illness like cancer. Ask a friend to come relieve you so you can spend some time taking care of yourself. Try to keep a normal schedule as much as possible, but this is going to require help from friends and family. It is normal for caregivers to get frustrated and feel like their patient doesn't understand the level of sacrifice they are making. Some hospitals offer support groups for caregivers. Ask your hospital's social worker about any resources they may offer. When William was first diagnosed, his doctor told us "taking care of William is going to be a full-time job for the next year or more." He was right! Doctor visits have ranged from one to five times a week, and the average time is six hours per visit. They also told us we had to avoid crowds while his immune system is compromised. This meant not going to church, shopping malls, or going out to eat at restaurants. Since we have younger children we had to heavily guard who they could play with. The doctor's preference was to completely eliminate William's contact with young children but since he had siblings who were two and four that wasn't possible. Even at family gatherings, I would wear a mask and gloves if there was a larger group or if anyone was coughing or sounded congested. I actually began to feel more comfortable with the mask on, than without it. I felt vulnerable without it. We had to wear masks while grocery shopping. It amused me how people would treat me in the grocery store when I was wearing a mask. They would cut a wide path around me, as if I were the one who was carrying some infectious disease, when in truth I was trying to protect myself from them. We also found it difficult to make any long-term plans. Things change in a second. William would be fine in the evening, and by morning he would be sitting in the emergency room. Always be flexible when making plans, and have a Plan B in the back of your mind because you never know what is going to happen from one minute to the next.

- Don't forget your spouse or partner. If you are caring for a parent or a child, and are in a relationship, don't be surprised if the two of you begin to argue. What happens is that you, the primary caregiver, are completely exhausted trying to care for your loved one and trying to keep up with your own daily routines and needs. You don't really have much energy or time to give to another person. Your partner begins to miss you, your old routine and the time you used to have together. He or she begins to get resentful and angry, not at you or the person you are caring for, but at the situation. When your partner tries to talk about it, it sounds like a verbal attack, and the fight is on! So many marriages end in divorce after a cancer diagnosis. Just like people, relationships can handle short-term stress, but cancer is a long-term stress, usually lasting several years. You need to be open in the beginning with your partner about this. Set expectations and boundaries. Go into it prepared, and make a game plan before the emotions get out of control. Early on, set a schedule for you and your spouse to get away from the house, just the two of you. Go out for dinner, see a movie or just go have a cup of coffee together.

Have a friend look after your loved one for you. While you are out, try not to talk about cancer, hospitals, insurance or anything medical. This is hard, because cancer consumes you and takes over every aspect of your life, but look for ways to connect with your spouse on a different level. Your partner is already resentful that cancer has consumed your lives; don't let it invade date night too. I didn't do this and I wish I had! It would have made this much easier on both of us, and probably cut out half our arguments. I would also suggest talking with a professional counselor. One day, we set an appointment for all of William's caregivers to talk with his counselor, Ted Graeser. Ted has been a big help for our family, and he even helped me with this section. He talked to each one of us about how we have handled the last year, and pointed out that each person handles grief differently, and William is handling it differently than each of us. Sometimes having someone to talk with that isn't so emotionally involved can really help diffuse a bad situation and also help open your eyes to how the other person is feeling. If your partner chooses not to see a counselor, I would still recommend that you go. Even alone you will still benefit greatly. Most insurance companies will cover professional counseling, and some hospitals offer the service for free. Ask your social worker to see what your hospital offers.

Glossary of Terms

These are some of the abbreviations and terms I have used throughout the book. The definitions provided are extremely basic, and not intended to give medical or treatment advice. For a more detailed explanation of any of these terms, consult with your health care professional.

- **Advanced Directives**, also called living wills, allow you to document your health care decisions regarding end-of-life treatment ahead of time. You may also be asked to give medical power of attorney to a trusted family member or friend, giving him or her legal authority to act on your behalf regarding your health care if you are not able to do so.

- **ALL- Acute Lymphoblastic Leukemia** is a rapidly progressing cancer of the white blood cells, called lymphocytes, in the bone marrow.

- **AML- Acute Myeloid Leukemia** is a rapidly progressing cancer of the myeloid stem cells in the bone marrow. Myeloid stem cells mature into red blood cells, white blood cells or platelets.

- **ANC- Absolute Neutrophil Count-** Neutrophils are a type of white blood cell that fights infections. These counts are usually lowered during the use of chemotherapy, making it difficult or impossible for the body to fight off infections.

- **AUL- Acute Undifferentiated Leukemia** is a rapidly progressing cancer that either shows markers of both ALL and AML, or the cells are so immature it is difficult to distinguish if the cancerous cells of the lymphocytes or myeloid lineage.

- **Blast Cells** refers to the percentage of immature cells found in bone marrow, the immature cells eventually grow to become red blood cells, white blood cells and platelets.

- **BMA- Bone Marrow Aspiration** is when a needle is inserted in the bone and a small amount of fluid and cells (bone marrow) is extracted.

- **BMT- Bone Marrow Transplant** is a procedure of replacing diseased or damaged bone marrow with healthy bone marrow collected from a donor. The donor is given general anesthesia and the cells are collected from the backside of the pelvic bone using a special syringe. The patient will undergo incredibly intense chemotherapy, and sometimes radiation to kill his or her own bone marrow to allow the new donor marrow to take over and produce healthy cells.

- **BMX- Bone Marrow Biopsy** is when a needle is inserted into the bone and a small amount of bone marrow (fluid and cells), as well as a small amount of the bone, are extracted.

- **Bolus-** an extra, or "breakthrough dose" of pain medication delivered from the PCA pump, usually administered by a nurse.

- **C DIFF- Clostridium difficile** is a contagious bacterial infection that causes diarrhea and colitis, which can range from mild to life-threatening. It typically occurs after using antibiotics for long periods of time, and is also commonly found in hospital or long term care facilities.

- **CMV-Cytomegalovirus** is a common virus most people have been exposed to and didn't realize it because symptoms are often "silent." Once infected, the body retains the virus for life but usually in healthy people it remains dormant. For those with a weakened immune system or pregnant women, it is a cause of concern.

- **CVC- Central Venous Catheter** is also called Subclavian Catheter or Central Line is a tube (or catheter) that is inserted into a large vein, usually in your chest, neck or groin, that is used for infusions and blood draws. It's basically a long-term IV that stays in you throughout your treatment.

- **DX-** an abbreviation usually referring to the date of a diagnosis

- **GVHD- Graft vs. Host Disease** is a condition in which the donor cells attack the host's body. The new cells do not recognize the host's cells, and see them as a foreign invader so their job is to attack and kill the invading cells. GVHD can show up in any area of the body, and should be treated right away, as it can be fatal if left untreated.

- **HGB-Hemoglobin** is the part of the red blood cells that carry oxygen to the body's tissues.

- **IVIG-** Intravenous Immunoglobulin is a blood product that contains antibodies from donated blood plasma. It is used to treat people with immune deficiencies and certain infections.

- **MDA-** MD Anderson Cancer Center in Houston, TX

- **Neutropenic** or neutropenia is a serious condition that makes the body vulnerable to catching infections of any kind. It happens when there is an abnormally low level of neutrophils in the blood (see ANC).

- **PCA Pump- Patient Controlled Analgesia Pump,** sometimes called a Morphine Pump, is a method of pain control that allows the patient to administer his or her own pain medication, through an IV by pushing a button. The doctor will set the limitations on how much and how often the medicine can be released.

- **PET Scan-Positron Emission Tomography** is a nuclear imaging technique used to diagnose several medical conditions, including cancer.

- **PICC Line- peripherally inserted central catheter** is the same as a CVC but inserted in the arm rather than the neck, chest or groin.

- **PLT- Platelets** are part of the blood that helps the blood clot.

- **SCT- Stem Cell Transplant** is a procedure of replacing diseased or damaged bone marrow with healthy stem cells collected from a donor. The donor takes medication to help his or her body produce more stem cells, and push them out into the blood stream. The cells are collected through the blood stream by inserting a sterile needle into one arm, allowing the blood to pass through a machine that separates and collects the stem cells and returns the blood to the donor through a needle in the other arm. The patient undergoes intensive chemotherapy, and sometimes radiation to kill his or her bone marrow, so that the new, transplanted, stem cells can produce healthy cells.

- **SSDI- Social Security Disability Insurance** pays benefits to you and certain members of your family if you are "insured," meaning that you worked long enough and paid Social Security taxes.

- **SSI- Supplemental Security Income** pays benefits based on financial need. If you have less than ten years of work history, you will not qualify for SSDI but still may receive SSI.

- **Stem Cells** are the immature cells that have the potential to develop into many different specialized cells. For the purpose of a bone marrow or stem cell transplant, stem cells can be taken from the bone marrow, circulating blood, or umbilical cords.

- **T-Cell** is a type of white blood cell that plays a key factor in the immune system.

- **VRE- Vancomycin resistant enterococci** is a type of bacterial infection that has developed resistance to Vancomycin and other antibiotics.

- **WBC- White Blood Cells** are cells the body makes to help fight infections.

FROM THE AUTHOR

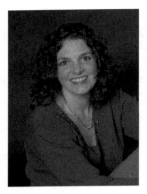

On June 6, 2103 at 10:34 p.m. I became a cancer mom. Before then, my life as a stay at home wife and mom was predictable and uneventful. But after my oldest son's leukemia diagnosis, my entire life changed. I have watched my son struggle through side effects of treatments that are nothing short of inhumane. I have buried friends, and hugged grieving moms and dads at the funerals of their children. I have studied statistics for survival rates, all the while wondering if my son was going to die. I have also seen the statistics of expected new cases, and they are rising at an alarming rate. I truly believe we need a cure, but we will never find the *cure* until we find the *cause*. Finding the cause of this disease takes funding. Therefore a portion of the proceeds from the sale of this book will be given to MD Anderson, Leukemia & Lymphoma Society and Leukemia Texas for both research and patient aid.

Until a cure is found, chemo and transplant are the best options we have. Since leukemia is a blood cancer, patients need constant blood and platelet transfusions to stay alive. So please, if your health allows it, become a regular blood donor at your local hospital or blood center. Those donations do save lives. Give, and give often.

Also join the national bone marrow registry. With 22 million registered donors, there was only ONE match for my son. Those are not good odds. The only way to better the odds is to add new donors. You can join for free at www.deletebloodcancer.org.

Join with me in the fight against this disease. Wouldn't it be amazing to see a cure in our lifetime!

Awareness=Funding. Funding=A Cure!

Amy Delaisse
Hope4William@gmail.com

101 - Nausea
145 Ansur
303"

Made in the USA
Middletown, DE
07 April 2024

52728672R00177